# PAIN-WISE

## A PATIENT'S GUIDE TO PAIN MANAGEMENT

DAVID KLOTH, M.D.
ANDREA TRESCOT, M.D.
FRANCIS RIEGLER, M.D.

*Pain-Wise*

Text Copyright © 2011 David Kloth, M.D., Andrea Trescot, M.D. and Francis Riegler, M.D.

Hatherleigh Press is committed to preserving and protecting the natural resources of the Earth. Environmentally responsible and sustainable practices are embraced within the company's mission statement.

Hatherleigh Press is a member of the Publishers Earth Alliance, committed to preserving and protecting the natural resources of the planet while developing a sustainable business model for the book publishing industry.

This book was edited and designed in the village of Hobart, New York. Hobart is a community that has embraced books and publishing as a component of its livelihood. There are several unique bookstores in the village. For more information, please visit www.hobartbookvillage.com.

Library of Congress Cataloging-in-Publication Data is available.
ISBN 978-1-57826-408-7

*Pain-Wise* is available for bulk purchase, special promotions, and premiums. For information on reselling and special purchase opportunities, call 1-800-528-2550 and ask for the Special Sales Manager.

Cover design by Nick Macagnone
Interior design by Nick Macagnone

10 9 8 7 6 5 4 3

Printed in the United States

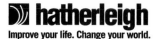

**hatherleigh**
Improve your life. Change your world.

# TABLE OF CONTENTS

# ACKNOWLEDGMENTS

The authors would like to thank Heather Gunnoud for her contributions to several chapters of this book and for her assistance in editing the early drafts of the manuscript.

# INTRODUCTION

So you've picked up this book, which likely means one of two things: either you are suffering from a condition that is causing **chronic pain**, or you are trying to understand the pain of a friend or loved one. We understand, and we're here to help. Pain management is one of the most misunderstood specialties, and it means many different things to different people. No doubt your head is swimming with all the treatment options being thrown at you. With so many options to choose from, you are probably wondering what exactly "pain management" is.

Pain management is a subspecialty of many different kinds of doctors. You can walk into the office of a doctor who promotes himself or herself as a pain management physician and see a psychiatrist, a **physiatrist**, a surgeon, an **anesthesiologist**, a **chiropractor**, an **acupuncturist**, or a variety of other physicians. In today's world, all of these different types of physicians may call themselves pain management doctors, and so this won't differentiate them from the more highly skilled and trained physicians who practice the subspecialty of **interventional pain management (IPM)**. Interventional pain physicians are experts at diagnosing and then treating chronic pain conditions using precision-guided injections or minimally invasive therapies. The types of physicians that may perform interventional pain management most commonly include anesthesiologists and physiatrists, but interventional pain management treatments are also performed by many other specialists, including radiologists, **neurologists, neurosurgeons, orthopedists,** and general practitioners. In some areas, a nurse practitioner or a physician assistant may perform these procedures (a practice which deeply concerns the authors of this book).

The complexity of different treatments and multitude of providers means that there is a great deal of variability in the level of training and quality of care. A patient, therefore, must become an active participant in his or her own care. You must be knowledgeable about your choices. Finding a doctor who will meet your needs and expectations requires at least as much research as buying a car. You wouldn't walk into a car dealership without knowing what kind of car you needed, what a reasonable price might be for that car, and what you should expect from your new vehicle. In the same way, you should walk into a pain management office knowing what type of doctor you're seeing, what his or her qualifications are, and what type of treatment you can expect. It is important that you understand the differences among providers so you can select the type of physician to best treat your particular pain problem.

The authors of this book strongly believe that the practice of interventional pain management is the practice of medicine and must only be performed by properly trained physicians and never by an independently practicing nurse or physician assistant. Interventional pain management physicians require extensive training to become proficient; the procedures are complex and can be very risky if not performed properly, so it is necessary that the physician has the proper background and training. The advice offered in this book comes from physicians who are actively practicing interventional pain management doctors. Interventional pain management is a specialty that focuses on determining the cause of symptoms and applying treatment options to manage and alleviate chronic pain. We are not simply generic "pain management" doctors. Interventional pain management physicians have a specific skill set, which will be explained in detail as this book progresses. We hope that this book will assist you in differentiating between the various interventional pain therapies and help guide you in both selecting a physician and learning about the various treatment options available today.

This book will begin with the basics and will then move to more complex concepts and treatments as it progresses. We have tried to include the more common treatments used today, but by no means is this meant to represent all possible therapies that are available. While we encourage you to read the whole book, please at least review the initial chapters which discuss important concepts that are relevant to all conditions (you may wish to use other parts of the book more as a reference). We encourage you to refer back to this book as you progress with treatment as we believe that you will find it to be a valuable resource as you work with your doctor to improve your pain and function.

**Note:**
All Glossary terms are marked in **bold** throughout the text for easy reference.

# CHAPTER 1

## A BRIEF HISTORY OF PAIN MEDICINE

Pain management or pain medicine is the branch of medicine devoted to the relief of pain and to improving the function and quality of life for those patients living in **chronic pain**. Although pain is a condition suffered by all creatures, the medical specialty of pain management is surprisingly new.

Perhaps the earliest reference to pain intervention is described in the book of Genesis in the Bible when God put Adam into a deep sleep in order to remove his rib to make Eve. Ancient cultures were well aware of the pain-relieving properties of plants; Egyptian papyrus records from 3000 BC described the use of poppy juice (opium) to treat pain. Chinese and other Eastern cultures identified pain points throughout the body and ultimately developed **acupuncture** therapy. Early Greek philosophers such as Plato recognized that the brain was the site of pain perception and showed its connection to the peripheral nervous system. In 1170 AD, the first book of Western surgery provides descriptions of sponges soaked in opium held over the patient's nose for surgical pain relief. Morphine was isolated from opium in 1806, the needle and syringe for hypodermic injections were developed in 1839, and ether was first used in 1846 to provide pain relief during surgery.

Cocaine, isolated from cocoa leaves from South America, was identified as a local anesthetic in 1860 and was used in nerve blocks soon afterwards. During the Civil War, which saw the first use of high-velocity bullets, physicians noticed that injury to nerves caused pain that seemed out of proportion to the injury itself. **Causalgia** (now known as **complex regional pain syndrome** type II), from the Greek word meaning "burning," was described by Weir-Mitchell in 1864.

1

In the late 19th century, using the newly developed hypodermic needles, cocaine and later pure alcohol were injected on nerves to provide pain relief during surgery, after injury, and for cancer patients. Novocain® (procaine), a local anesthetic that is not addictive, does not cause euphoric effects, and is not related to cocaine, was developed in 1904. World War I (1914 to 1918) and World War II (1939 to 1945) provided ample opportunity to use this new knowledge to treat pain. Patients suffering from trauma, frostbite, and **phantom-limb pain**, as well as neuropathic pain syndromes like causalgia, underwent injections of the safer local anesthetics that by then had largely replaced cocaine.

It was during World War II that an army surgeon by the name of John Bonica started a multidisciplinary approach to pain management on veterans with chronic pain, which drew attention to the under-treatment of pain in general and chronic pain in particular. His intellectual approach and organized medicine efforts, as well as his 1953 publication of the first comprehensive book on pain management, *The Management of Pain,* led to his universally recognized role in history as the founder of modern pain management. John Bonica worked at the University of Washington in Seattle after World War II, and his efforts inspired the founding of the International Association for the Study of Pain (IASP) in 1973 and the American Pain Society (APS) in 1977.

By the late 1980s, it became clear that pain could be treated not only by oral medications but also by the delivery of specific medications to specific structures via injection. In medicine, there are radiologists who look at x-rays and interventional radiologists who use x-rays to direct needles to specific structures to obtain tissue for diagnosis; there are **cardiologists** who read EKGs and prescribe blood pressure medicines and interventional cardiologists who use **catheterization** and x-rays to open up blood vessels and insert stents. Borrowing that concept, in 1990 Steve Waldman coined the term **"interventional pain management"** to distinguish medication management of pain from injection therapy. The first textbook on interventional pain, *Interventional Pain Management* by Steven Waldman and Alon Winnie, was published in 1995. Early in the field's development, the majority of physicians choosing to specialize in pain management were anesthesiologists and most training programs are still under the auspices of anesthesia departments. Because of this history, the American Society of Anesthesiologists (ASA) has played a large role in this field and many of the interventional pain management techniques being used today were developed by anesthesiologists. By the late 1990s, many anesthesiologists began to leave the practice of operative anesthesia and focus instead on full-time interventional pain medicine. At around the same time, doctors from other specialties such as radiology, neurology, and physical medicine and rehabilitation also began to practice full-time interventional pain medicine.

The American Academy of Pain Medicine (AAPM) was established in 1985 as a multi-specialty physician pain society. The International Spine Intervention Society (ISIS) was established in 1993 as an association of physicians interested in the development, implementation, and standardization of **percutaneous** (delivered through the skin) techniques with precision diagnosis of spinal pain. In 1998, the American Society of Interventional Pain Physicians (ASIPP) was formed to preserve, advance, and promote the development and practice of safe, high-quality, and cost-effective IPM techniques.

The American Board of Anesthesiologists (ABA) gave the first specialty certification examination in pain medicine to anesthesiologists in 1993; the American Board of Pain Medicine (ABPM) began to administer a pain board certification available to multiple specialties in 1995. The United States Congress established the specialty designation of interventional pain management, separate from anesthesia, in 2003.

In 2006, the American Board of Interventional Pain Physicians (ABIPP) developed a board certification specifically for interventional pain physicians, which includes a written exam, an oral exam, and a practical exam (on a cadaver) to evaluate the various components of a pain physician's training. ABIPP also tests for training in the proper use and management of controlled substances as well as practice management as it relates to rules, regulations, and billing activities. Today, this stands as the most comprehensive exam for testing interventional pain physicians.

In June of 2011, the Institute of Medicine, a federal agency, released a legislatively commissioned report which describes the massive economic impact of chronic pain which costs this nation more than heart disease in medical bills, sick days, and lost productivity. The report also comments on the barriers to accessing proper pain management therapies which include inadequate research, insurance that does not cover complex care, and health workers not adequately trained to handle pain issues.

While it is true that virtually every patient who visits a doctor complains of pain, specialty training and certification in pain medicine is really barely 20 years old—a youngster when compared to the specialties of internal medicine or surgery. Hopefully, all physicians will someday be required to undergo training in pain medicine prior to graduation from medical school. Until then, it is important for patients to understand the training and credentials of their potential pain physician.

When looking for a physician, you may find that some specialize in one or more aspects of pain treatment. Some may just prescribe medications, some just do injections, some may do counseling, others only manipulate parts of the body, and others will provide a combination of these approaches. We suggest that you select a physician who has the proper training and background for the care that you require, and who dedicates at least 50% of his or her professional practice to the treatment of pain. It is important to understand what services your doctor can provide and whether he or she works with other doctors or health care professionals who offer other components of pain management so that you have access to the full spectrum of pain care.

# CHAPTER 2

## NOT ALL PAIN PHYSICIANS ARE THE SAME

If you or a loved one suffers from **chronic pain**, you're probably wary of seeing yet another doctor. In the search for pain relief, the true pain specialist usually is not consulted until the patient has exhausted every other option, including practitioners of other disciplines that often market themselves as "pain specialists," such as **chiropractors** and massage therapists. Many patients—and unfortunately, even many doctors—do not understand the difference between the different types of pain providers. This is surprising and not necessarily the way it should be, but this is the way it is for most patients.

All too often patients are told that everything that can be done for their problem has been done. But they still have unrelieved pain. Patients are often told other treatment alternatives are too risky or are unlikely to help them. If the doctor can't figure out what is causing the pain, he or she may begin to think the patient is making up the symptoms for secondary gain (money, insurance, drugs, etc.), or the doctor may take what has become the easy way out and diagnose the pain as fibromyalgia. Although fibromyalgia is a real condition, it has recently become a catch-all diagnosis for patients with pain that isn't easily explained, and some doctors find it easier to attach this label than look for what might be a treatable cause of pain.

The most important part of any pain treatment is making the right diagnosis. How can you treat the problem if you don't know what is wrong? For instance, taking out the appendix may be a great surgery for belly pain, unless the problem is your gall bladder. Pain that persists beyond a reasonable period of time and continues despite some initial treatment will likely require more precise evaluation by a physician who specializes in the diagnosis and treatment of pain. Pain

5

specialists have been trained to find the specific cause of pain by using your history, physical findings, various radiologic and laboratory studies, and often specific and highly targeted injections to determine the exact cause of your pain.

The answer is rarely just to take another pill or to increase the current medications; rather, it is best to identify and treat the specific underlying cause. Your bank account also probably needs help, because you have spent yourself silly trying everything else along the way. By this point, the pain has likely also affected your work, or perhaps you haven't been able to work because of the pain. Pain can have a dramatically negative effect on normal activities and can limit many aspects of life that you enjoy. Chronic pain also often causes moodiness and depression, which are real consequences for your mental health and which will affect your interactions with others.

You are in pain, tired, frustrated, poorer, angry, and suspicious of "yet another doctor," so you need to make sure that, if you are going to make the effort to see a pain specialist, it is someone who is competent and appropriate for your problem. But it is often not as easy as checking the Yellow Pages under "pain specialist." Unfortunately, sometimes you don't have a choice of doctors because your insurance company limits your choices, or your regular medical doctor may not know where to direct you for this highly specialized care.

Within the next few pages, we will explore the differences between different kinds of doctors who specialize in pain management so that you can find a doctor who can help you figure out the cause of your symptoms and develop an effective treatment plan to help control or manage the pain. You will note that we did not use the word "cure," as this may or may not be an achievable goal, depending on your particular condition (for more about managing expectations, see chapter 3).

## Choosing the Right Physician for Your Problem

At the beginning of this book, you learned that interventional pain physicians can come from different specialty backgrounds. That is because **interventional pain management** is a "hybrid" specialty that developed from various other specialties. Unfortunately, IPM is such a new field that there isn't a specific residency training program that targets this medical specialty, so all physicians who work in the pain field have gone through training in another field of medicine first. Today, if a bright young medical student wants to practice IPM, he or she has to do an internship, then a residency in another specialty, and only then can he or she can finally do formal training in IPM through a fellowship or post-residency training.

Some physicians have been practicing pain management so long that their training predates formal fellowships, which have only existed since the early 1990s. Some clinicians entered IPM later in their career via a different specialty. Some of these clinicians have had proper training, and others call themselves specialists merely because they have attended a weekend course or two. Unfortunately, many physicians claim to be pain specialists (or attempt to perform pain procedures) despite the lack of any formal training in this field of medicine. The true pain specialist has spent extensive time studying this complex and rapidly evolving specialty. In fact, the work is so specific and the developments so rapid that it is the rare physician who can split his or her time between performing IPM and working in another area of medical practice.

Besides asking about formal training in pain management, you can check what board certifications your physician holds. This will give you information about their level, and type, of training. It is important to understand the different types of board certifications that are available for pain doctors. The most rigorous of these examinations is also perhaps one of the most intensive and in-depth examination processes in medicine today. This exam was developed by the American Society of Interventional Pain Physicians (ASIPP), a specialty society of physicians practicing IPM. Once the physician passes this examination, he or she becomes a "diplomate" of the American Board of Interventional Pain Physicians (ABIPP).

So what else is out there? The only certification officially accepted by the American Board of Medical Specialties (ABMS) at this time is the American Board of Anesthesiologists (ABA) "certificate of added qualifications" in pain management. The ABA gave its first examination in 1993. Now two other specialties—physical medicine and rehabilitation (PM&R) and neurology/psychiatry—are allowed to take the same examination. This exam tests for general knowledge in a variety of areas of pain medicine but does not thoroughly test the IPM physician's knowledge of interventional techniques. Today, the number of **anesthesiologists** with pain certification is much greater than the other fields. That is partly because anesthesiologists originally were the only ones who could take the examination and also because anesthesiologists were the first specialists to provide the injection treatments that are part of IPM today.

However, a certificate of added qualifications doesn't actually certify physicians to perform IPM; rather, it tests only their general pain knowledge. This is important too, and so is still required as the first part of the ABIPP exam, but it doesn't adequately test physicians' practical and technical proficiency in IPM. Nevertheless, this was the closest thing to certification in pain management until just a few years ago. That's when the American Board of Interventional Pain Physicians (ABIPP) was formed to more properly and fully test the IPM specialist. At around the same time, the World Institute of Pain (WIP), an international organization, began giving oral and practical (cadaver) exams in IPM to establish clinical and technical proficiency in IPM. Those who completed the examination process were awarded a Fellow of Interventional Pain Practice (FIPP) certificate. Working with WIP, ABIPP initially used this certification to count toward the second part of the ABIPP exam, but ABIPP recently developed their own format for this portion of the examination process. ABIPP has two other important components to its examination process: a test on controlled substance management and another on compliance, documentation, and coding.

You can see that a physician who is certified by ABIPP is a rare physician who has gone through an extremely intensive board examination process that includes at least five written exams, an oral exam, and a practical exam that requires the applicant to demonstrate his or her clinical skills on a cadaver in front of two examiners. If your doctor is ABIPP certified, he or she is one of the few physicians willing to prove their skill as an interventional pain physician. ABIPP is not yet a Member Board of the American Board of Medical Specialties. ABMS is the oldest and most prestigious organization of medical specialty boards. Pain management has a toehold at ABMS via the certificates issued by certain member boards. But ABIPP hopes to elevate pain management to the level of having its own board.

If you have an ABIPP-certified pain doctor, then you can feel confident that you've found someone who has the skill and knowledge to help you with your chronic pain. But what if you can't find someone who is ABIPP certified? Unfortunately, that is going to be the usual circumstance for at least a few more years. Today, there are less than 500 ABIPP certified doctors, but bear in mind this is a new process; hopefully, the numbers will continue to grow.

So how do you know if a specific doctor has the skills to help you? There are a couple of ways to size up your doctor. First of all, don't be afraid to ask questions. Here are some key criteria, listed in order of importance, to help you evaluate your physician:

- *Certification.* Does the doctor hold a certificate in pain management from any board? You can go to the American Board of Medical Specialties (ABMS) website (www.abms.org) to see if your doctor is ABMS certified and if they hold a specialty certificate in pain management from an ABMS member board. If you want to confirm that your doctor has an ABIPP certificate, check their website (www.abipp.org).

- *Training.* Where did the doctor do his or her residency? In what specialty? Did he or she do a fellowship in pain management?

- *Level of involvement.* Ideally, your doctor practices pain management or IPM full time.

- *Credentials.* Does your doctor have credentials at a local hospital or surgery center to practice interventional pain management? You can easily check with the hospital or local surgery center. Credentialing is different from board certification, but if a hospital or surgical center has granted the physician privileges, they have theoretically checked at least for basic competence—although we caution you that this may not always be the case. It is still possible in certain places to get credentials to practice IPM without being board certified or even properly trained.

- *Experience.* How long has the doctor been practicing IPM—not just practicing medicine but practicing pain management in general and IPM in particular? Is his or her whole practice dedicated to pain management, or does he or she just dabble in the field? Given the complexity of this field, a true pain physician should dedicate at least 50% of their professional time to practicing pain management.

- *Society membership and meeting attendance.* One of the ways that doctors stay current in their field is to attend meetings where they can learn and network with other doctors in their specialty. Because IPM is a rapidly changing field, it is critical for your doctor to stay current, and the societies and meetings are a good source of new information.

- *Peer recommendation.* Your other physicians may be able to give you a referral to a physician who specializes in pain management. Unfortunately, this may be the least reliable method, because some referring physicians may not understand the differences in pain medicine training that we discussed earlier.

# CHAPTER 3

## WHAT TO EXPECT FROM INTERVENTIONAL PAIN MANAGEMENT

**C**hronic pain, back problems, neck problems, disc **degeneration,** headaches, and pelvic pain are all identifiable diseases and must be treated as such. The goal of **interventional pain management** procedures should be to reduce and manage pain, with emphasis on the word "manage." Your physician may not necessarily be able to cure the problem, but they can help you control the pain and maximize your functional level. Although the ideal goal may be to completely resolve the issue and the associated pain, this is often not realistically possible. This is also true for the majority of other chronic health problems. When the **pancreas** does not secrete **insulin,** patients are diagnosed with diabetes and treated with insulin for the rest of their lives; chronic heart conditions are treated on an ongoing basis with heart medications, and so on. Chronic pain similarly may require intermittent or continual treatment. When patients have bad **discs** that are severely degenerated and then develop chronic back pain, they will likely require intermittent treatment for the rest of their life. It is important to have a conversation with your pain physician so that you can ask him or her to explain what can and cannot be achieved with a particular injury or degree of damage. And don't let anyone tell you that surgery will cure; even when it fixes what it intends, it can cause significant problems to adjacent structures. This is true if it is your back or knee (or any body part).

While some conditions can be cured, most are managed to provide long-term control. Realistic expectations are extremely important and should be agreed upon in advance with your doctor. If a patient expects to be 100 % cured and this does not occur, he or she will obviously be disappointed. If the doctor's and the patient's expectations are radically different, neither will be satisfied with the outcome. When both parties are trying to achieve a 50% to 70% reduction in pain and that goal is reached, both parties will be happy. The role of the pain management physician is often to manage the pain as completely as possible while recognizing that all the pain may not be eliminated.

So when is enough treatment enough? The answer is actually quite simple: when you reach a point where the pain level is tolerable. This varies from patient to patient. In a successful outcome, pain only minimally interferes with the activities of daily living, and symptoms are adequately controlled with either no medication or very low dosages. It is often difficult to determine when the patient is as good as he or she is going to get and when to stop performing procedures. We frequently see patients whose backs and discs are damaged so severely that we have limited options to control the symptoms. For example, patients who have had multiple previous surgeries or who have multilevel damage rarely respond to further surgery. In these situations, we try to control the acute problems, the most severe pain, and then control other remaining symptoms until they're tolerable.

In this book, we have provided you with a basic understanding of the various treatment options that exist today for both diagnosing and treating pain. There are many options available to relieve chronic pain, but they all rely on first finding the correct diagnosis. Don't be afraid to ask your doctor questions that they may not have covered. Finding the right physician with the proper training is a great start. Going through the proper diagnostic evaluations and procedures will help to identify the specific causes of your pain. Although your pain physicians will likely not promise you 100% relief, they should offer to help reduce your pain, improve your functioning, and help you return to a more normal daily life.

## Before Your First Appointment:

1. Complete any paperwork the doctor requires. Many practices have lengthy questionnaires for new patients, and you may be asked to fill one out before you can be seen. Take your time and answer the questions thoughtfully. Some of the questions may seem irrelevant, but your answers help the doctor to understand your problem and how it affects your life, and to determine what treatments are most suitable for you.

2. Bring the results from any MRI or **CT scans** you have had. These results include a written report from the radiologist who originally read the scan as well as a copy of the pictures themselves. These pictures can be actual films or on CD. In many cases, your pain management physician needs to see these pictures before he or she can come up with a treatment plan. You will save yourself time if you bring the films to your first appointment. The saying "a picture is worth a thousand words" is also true in evaluating your condition.

3. Bring your insurance card and picture ID.

4. Make sure that you understand your insurance plan and how much you will be expected to pay at your first visit. For most people, this will mean that you will need to pay a copay. Be prepared to make this payment. If you don't carry cash, make sure the office takes checks or credit cards.

5. If your insurance plan requires a primary-care physician referral, make sure one is in place.

6. Wear comfortable clothing that is easy to remove. During your first visit, a neurologic exam may be performed. For example, if you have back pain that radiates into your legs, testing may be done on your legs and feet. Wear shoes that come off easily to make the experience easier for you.

7. Bring any relevant medical records. If another physician sent you to the pain management office, that physician should have sent all the necessary records. Trust but verify: check to make sure the records arrived in advance; if they have not, do your best to obtain all relevant records and bring them with you to your first appointment.

## Before Any Procedure:

1. Make your doctor aware of all medications you're taking. Some heart medications are **blood thinners** and will increase the risk of bleeding complications.

2. If you are diabetic, you must tell your physician ahead of time. Insulin-dependent diabetics will have to follow specific protocols before and after any injection. If you are having your procedure with sedation, you will need to fast before the procedure, and you should bring your insulin with you to the procedure. Steroids can increase your blood sugar and so you may need to work with

your diabetic doctor to adjust your dosages as indicated.

3. Because some procedures require sedation, you must not eat or drink for several hours before the procedure, because when you are sedated you are more likely to inhale food and stomach acid into the lungs, which can result in severe pneumonia.

# CHAPTER 4

---

# ANATOMY: AN EXPLANATION OF THE PARTS OF YOU THAT YOU CAN'T SEE IN THE MIRROR

You may be tempted to skip this chapter because you think that it is going to be very complex or way too much like high school biology. We have tried to make this easy to understand. People tend to know more about their cars than they do about their own bodies, but the patient in pain needs to understand why his or her body is hurting to understand how to get better. This section will help you to understand some of the procedures that are discussed in later sections. If you decide to skip this chapter (and even if you don't), we urge you to refer back to these pages to better understand the anatomy of the region we are discussing. If it seems boring, read only the parts that apply to your problem. You can always come back and read the other sections when you can't sleep at night.

## The Central Nervous System

The spine and **central nervous system** are the key to understanding pain. These complex structures are literally the "backbone" of most pain treatments. As **degeneration** and damage occurs to structures of the spine, various parts of the nervous system are affected, including the spinal cord and nerve roots as they travel down from the brain and then exit the **spinal canal**. The spinal canal is the cylindrical tube that runs from the base of the brain to the tailbone. This is where the spinal cord is located and where the nerve roots exit to travel to all the other parts of the body (figure 4.1).

Pain is processed through nerve endings called receptors and then transmitted through nerves into the spinal cord; messages are sent from the spinal cord to the brain, which you then perceive as the sensation of pain. Different structures and types of injuries produce different qualities or sensations of pain. For example, burning pain typically accompanies damage to nerves and aching pain is commonly associated with muscular and/or skeletal injuries. Processing these inputs into the central nervous system (brain and spinal cord) leads to the conscious perception of pain. Manipulation of this same process also allows us to treat pain and/or change the patient's perception of pain.

Interventional pain treatments are typically directed at areas where nerves are being irritated, compressed, or damaged. Irritation can come from direct compression from a protruding disc (figure 4.2) and/or from a bone or ligament overgrowth (figures 4.3 a, b, and c). It can also be caused by chemical irritation from a **leaking disc**. The bony structures of the spine guide the placement of the interventional pain physician's needles. Using fluoroscopic or x-ray guidance, the physician injects structures or areas within the spine that are the cause of pain. Occasionally, physicians will use a **CAT scan** (now more commonly called a **CT scan**) or **ultrasound** for guidance. Each of these methods has advantages and disadvantages. Most physicians will use a rotating x-ray machine called a **C-arm**; because of its curved shape, it moves in multiple different directions allowing the doctor to get real-time images without moving the patient. With this machine, the physician can view the bony structures from many different angles and determine their relationship to the needle, which allows precision-guided placement of the injection.

Several structures within the spine are typical injection sites. For instance, the **epidural space** is the space between the spinal cord and the bony spinal canal (figure 4.4). The spinal nerves pass through this space to leave the spinal canal, and medication in the epidural space placed near a nerve that is being compressed or irritated can relieve pain. These injections are typically referred to as epidural steroid injections, which can actually describe a variety of different injection techniques (see chapter 10).

By convention, physicians separate the spine into four specific areas (see figure 4.1): cervical (neck), thoracic (mid-back), lumbar (low back), and sacral (buttock). There are seven **cervical vertebra bones**, labeled C1 to C7. There are also 12 thoracic vertebral bones, labeled T1 to T12, and five **lumbar vertebral bones**, labeled L1 to L5. The sacrum is composed of five fused vertebrae (although some patients have more or less vertebrae, which are known as

**transitional segments**). The **coccyx**, or tailbone, is usually a fused collection of three smaller bones. Each spinal level, or vertebral body, is separated from the next by a disc in the front of the spine and a set of paired joints in the back of the spine called facets (figure 4.5).

There are two specially named vertebral bodies: the **atlas** (C1), on which the skull rests; and the **axis** (C2), which is shaped sort of like a post on which the atlas sits and rotates. The joints located between C1 and C2 are called the **atlanto-axial (AA) joints**. The **atlanto-occipital (AO) joints** are located between the occiput and C1. These paired joints basically run from the skull to the base of the spine and are oriented in different directions, or planes, in different areas of the spine (for example, the neck or the back); they are prone to specific injuries depending on the direction and type of force applied. Each joint has multiple nerves that go to it, one set at that level and one set from the level above (figure 4.6).

Any one of these paired joints on either or both sides can cause pain. Arthritic degeneration or traumatic injury such as a whiplash phenomenon or twisting injury can cause pain in **facet joints** within the spine and/or **sacroiliac joints** in the pelvis. Like the facet joints, the sacroiliac joints are paired structures on each side of the body (figure 4.7). Sacroiliac joint injuries can lead to instability of the joint in addition to pain. Slips and falls or a traumatic event such as a car accident can make these joints unstable and cause them to slip in and out of position (figure 4.8).

Nerves can be compressed by a **disc herniation**, collapse of the disc, or bone overgrowth and degeneration. The disc is the soft tissue—the shock absorber—between each bone of the spine; these **discs** can protrude or bulge backward into the spinal canal, pushing on a nerve (figure 4.2) and causing pain. Nerves can also be compressed or pinched by bony overgrowths caused by arthritic changes and by too much motion of the spine, referred to as instability. As the spine ages, the joints compensate for the ongoing stressors of life by growing larger to better support the spine. Some of the **ligaments** or other supporting structures of the spine can also thicken (**hypertrophy**). The combination of these factors can lead to narrowing of the central spinal canal where the nerves travel, called **spinal stenosis**. Stenosis can occur centrally or in the holes where the nerves exit (the **neural foramen**) (figures 4.3 a, b, and c). This can cause compression of the nerves, which causes secondary inflammation of the nerve and causes pain. Steroid injections can reverse or treat this inflammatory process and decrease pain, but injections won't change the underlying anatomy. While surgery can certainly change the underlying anatomy, and sometimes this really helps, surgery can sometimes also lead to its own set of problems.

After the nerves exit the spinal canal, they gather into major nerve trunks going to both the arms (**brachial plexus**) and legs (the **sciatic nerve**). In the chest and abdomen as well as in the arms and legs, these trunks then break into **peripheral nerves** (those outside the spinal column). Nerves can be damaged anywhere along their course by traumatic injuries, radiation, or surgery. Injuries to the nerves anywhere along their course can cause the development of a particularly severe type of pain syndrome, typically referred to as a **complex regional pain syndrome (CRPS)**, which is discussed further in chapter 18.

### Transitional Segments: How Many Bones In Your Lumbar Spine?

Approximately 7% of the American population and approximately 15% of patients with chronic lower back pain have what is called a transitional segment of the spine (figure 4.9). In this congenital abnormality (that is, a condition present at birth), the bones in the lumbar spine and pelvis are altered, either by being born with one too many or one too few bones in the lumbar spine and therefore fewer or more discs. Although there may be no pain involved with these "design flaws" (one of the authors of this book has a transitional vertebra without any pain), it appears that patients with this abnormality are more prone to the development of chronic lower back pain; twice the percentage of people with chronic back pain have this finding compared to the regular population. It is important that doctors recognize this abnormality as it can have a significant bearing on treatment outcomes. Also, because nerves exit and work on very specific areas, knowing which nerve is most likely to be affected is important for proper treatment.

# CHAPTER 5

## DIAGNOSTIC TESTING: RADIOLOGY AND ELECTRODIAGNOSTIC MEDICINE

You have probably already had your share of radiologic tests and are wondering if you are going to start glowing in the dark. It's very common to be concerned about the level of radiation you are being exposed to, but keep in mind that not every test done by a radiologist involves exposure to radiation (for instance MRIs use magnets, not radiation, to develop an image of the body's internal structures). Patients who should be most concerned about radiation exposure are women who are, or may be, pregnant. If you think it is possible that you are pregnant, please make sure you tell the doctor ordering your test and the doctor performing the test before it is done.

Each test plays an important and specific role in determining what part of the body or anatomical structure may be contributing to your pain and will help your doctor to diagnose and figure out how to treat your problem. The part of the body and makeup of the structure (whether it's bone or soft tissue) will help form your doctor's decisions about which tests to perform for the best assessment of the area in question. Think of these tests like different types of eye glasses; you choose different glasses to see different things in specific conditions. If it's sunny out, you wear sunglasses. You might wear reading glasses to read a book. If you need to see something really far away, you might use binoculars, and if you're looking even farther away, you might use a telescope. When your doctor selects a test, he or she is considering what needs to be seen and the best way to see it.

## Radiology: A Look Inside the Body

When patients begin treatment, they often have simple x-rays of the traumatized area. For example, if you had a slip or fall that landed you in the emergency room, it is very likely that an x-ray would have been taken to make sure no bones were broken. Simple x-rays are very good for looking at bones and can also help diagnose some conditions, such as arthritis (figure 5.1). Different angles and views may be obtained to better see the part of the body in question. Occasionally, x-rays are taken in various positions (for instance, leaning forward and then bending backwards) to see if the bones are moving in relation to each other and to assess the degree of instability. Sometimes fractures are so subtle that it becomes difficult to see them on x-ray and more specialized testing is required.

The next most common test that people with spine-related problems will have is magnetic resonance imaging (MRI). MRI (figures 5.2 a and b) does not involve the use of radiation; it uses strong magnetic fields to look at soft-tissue structures within the body. Some soft tissue structures may appear on x-rays and **CT scans**, but MRI provides the best look at this type of structure. MRI scans are often the main diagnostic test ordered when there is a concern about a **disc herniation** because **discs** are made of soft tissue, not bone. MRI can look at bones as well. In fact, MRI can be a very helpful tool when looking at bones because it shows the inflammation or **edema** from a recent fracture or from chronic instability/excessive motion. MRI scans provide multiple views of an area that can help provide clearer pictures of certain structures.

Sometimes contrast is given during an MRI scan. The contrast is given by vein so that it will flow with your blood to different parts of the body. Pictures are taken before and after the contrast is injected. If a patient has had surgery, the scar tissue will "light up" on the MR images. This helps the radiologist and your doctor differentiate between what is scar tissue and what may be a recurrent disc herniation. MRI can also be very helpful to identify tears or cracks in the outer wall of the disc, a defect that is commonly associated with back pain.

Sometimes, your doctor will send you for a CT scan (figure 5.3). This is also called a **CAT scan**, which stands for computed axial tomography. CT scans are typically used for bony structures. CT scans are also combined with other radiology tests such as **discograms** and **myelograms** to better see the dye that has been injected into the spine. During discography (see chapter 16), dye is injected into the disc; a CT scan, which typically follows the discogram, can then help doctors visualize the exact location where the disc is leaking. CT scans are also done after myelograms (injections of dye into the spinal fluid) to better tell which nerve roots are compressed. By looking for areas where the dye doesn't flow, doctors can find areas where there is nerve compression.

Nuclear medicine scans involve labeling normal cells within the body using various radioactive isotopes, and then following those cells to see if they lead us to the problem (this is very safe, even though it sounds like something scary out of a sci-fi movie). This can be used to find hidden fractures or infections in a bone or other deep cavity of the body. Stress tests for the heart commonly include a nuclear medicine scan.

One of the more common types of nuclear medicine study is a **bone scan,** which is used to follow metabolic changes in the bone as a sign of hidden fractures, infection, or tumor. Often these findings are not associated with major radiologic changes (figure 5.4). Bone scans can also check for fusion healing (after surgery) and bone inflammation, such as occurs with arthritis. Bone scans will show increased uptake or changes in areas of acute inflammation and increased bone activity. Bone scans are also sometimes used for evaluation of **complex regional pain syndrome** (CRPS, see chapter 18) and will show different findings during the various stages of the disease. Many patients (about a third) will not show bone changes despite having the diagnosis of CRPS. Therefore, this particular test does not necessarily rule out a diagnosis of CRPS but can help to confirm it.

Other more specific tests, such as positron emission tomography (PET) scans, are commonly used in the evaluation of cancer. This particular test looks for increased metabolic activity. Cancer is associated with an overgrowth of abnormal cells in the body, which is seen as increased metabolic activity due to the rapid growth that occurs in the area of a tumor. When areas of higher metabolic activity are seen on a PET scan, it may tell your doctor where the disease may have spread. PET scans are also used to see if the cancer is responding to treatment.

If you have back or neck pain, it is likely that your doctor will either review tests that you have already had or send you for more tests during the workup and treatment of your condition. These tests are extremely important in helping your doctor determine the exact cause of your pain and also in helping him or her treat your symptoms. Make sure you know where all of your test results are, and bring them with you to your first appointment, if possible. If you have already had an MRI, your physician may not need to order another MRI. If you have had an MRI in the past and your physician orders a new one, it is often helpful to compare the two scans to see what has changed.

Once your doctor has seen the complete picture from all of these tests, it will be easier to make the right diagnosis and get you feeling better. Also, remember that your doctor may not have the results of your testing right away. Some tests give immediate results but other tests may take more time to get the results. For example, MRI images and CT scans are made up of hundreds of individual pictures that a radiologist has to interpret. The radiologist will prepare a report based on what he or she sees in the pictures and will then send a copy to the doctor who referred you for the test. Your doctor will usually want to see your actual films, so check with your doctor's office to see if you should bring copies of the study to your next appointment.

## Questions to Ask Your Doctor:

1. Ask your doctor if he would like you to bring copies of any tests to your next appointment. In addition to getting a report from the radiologist, some doctors like to review the pictures from MRI, CT scans, and x-rays themselves. These pictures are made on large pieces of plastic that are viewed on light boxes or on CDs that are viewed on computers.

2. Ask your doctor when he would like you to come back to the office to discuss the results. Depending on the type of test and what will be done with the information, your doctor may want to send you for additional testing or see you in the office first to discuss the next step in your treatment plan.

3. Ask your doctor if your insurance carrier requires precertification for the tests you are about to undergo. If you need precertification, find out who will be contacting you to schedule the test. If you schedule your own test and it needs to be authorized first, you may be stuck with a rather large bill. Once your test is scheduled, if you change the date of your test or the facility where you are having it done, let your doctor's office know ahead of time. Many insurance carriers require that your doctor's office tell them ahead of time where you are having your scan. If you go

somewhere else, the approval may no longer be valid and then you will possibly be responsible again for the cost of the test.

## Before the Procedure:

1. MRI machines use high-powered magnets. If you have any metal in your body, tell your doctor and the radiologist *before* you undergo the test. Metal in your body may include screws, rods, and artificial joints. It also includes implants for chronic pain management (see chapter 20). If you have ever worked with metal (welders, etc.), you may need to undergo an x-ray before the MRI to make sure you don't have any slivers of metal lodged under your skin or in your eyes.

2. If there is any chance that you are pregnant or may become pregnant, discuss this with your doctor before undergoing any testing. The decision to do the test may require a conversation between your pain doctor and your obstetrician. Sometimes you will need to have a radiology test even if you are pregnant. Some tests are relatively safe for your unborn baby.

3. Make sure your doctor is aware of any surgery you may have had in the past. For instance, if you have had prior back surgery, you will need to have contrast or dye with your MRI.

4. Tell your physician if you have any issues with claustrophobia. Claustrophobia is the fear of being in an enclosed space. MRI machines are essentially large tubes that your body is placed in, and if you are claustrophobic, you may need to take some medication ahead of time to make sure this experience is as comfortable as possible.

## Electrodiagnostic Medicine: More Tests to Complete the Picture

When you first see an interventional pain physician, you will undergo a history, physical examination, and appropriate testing. In many cases, you might have an MRI or a CT scan as part of your workup. However, sometimes additional specialized testing might be warranted. Physicians refer to this kind of testing as electrodiagnosis. This information gives the doctor a better idea of how certain nerves and muscles in the body may be affected by your condition. The information obtained from **electrodiagnostic testing** will help determine a more precise diagnosis.

For example, if you have pain in your lower back and one or both of your legs, a properly conducted history, physical examination, and MRI result might all point to some degenerated discs in your lumbar spine. Electrodiagnostic testing can help determine which particular disc level(s) need treatment. In that case, your pain physician can more precisely focus the treatment at the affected disc level(s). If you experience pain and numbness in your arm and hand, there are at least two locations where this problem could be coming from: your neck or your wrist. Electrodiagnostics can help focus the diagnosis, and thereby direct the physician to the more appropriate treatment.

Electrodiagnostic testing is usually done by a physician with a background in neurology or physical medicine and rehabilitation. In some cases, your interventional pain physician may perform the test if he or she has that specialty background. Some physicians are certified by the American Board of Electrodiagnostic Medicine (ABEM), but this is rarely mandated.

## Nerve Conduction Study and Electromyography

One of the more frequently performed sets of tests is a **nerve conduction study (NCS)** and **electromyography (EMG)**. Having an EMG or a nerve conduction study for your nerves and muscles is like having an electrocardiogram (ECG) for your heart.

A nerve conduction study evaluates the speed and number of nerve fibers that are working. The test allows your doctor to determine how the nerves are functioning. By measuring the speed at which an impulse travels and the appearance of wave forms, they can determine the type and extent of nerve injury. Just like with an ECG, there are normal waveforms and abnormal waveforms. Abnormal waveforms suggest the source of the problem. These measurements are compared from one side of the body to the other, and also against published and standardized data obtained from thousands of patients. The activation of the stimulator used during the test feels like static electricity, such as when you rub your feet on a carpet and then touch another person. One portion of this test is done by inserting a needle into the muscles, which can be uncomfortable but is not usually painful.

# CHAPTER 6

## COMPREHENSIVE PAIN THERAPY: OTHER PIECES OF THE PUZZLE

**I**nterventional **pain management** treatments are rarely performed in isolation and are usually combined with physical therapy and other therapeutic treatment modalities. As a general principle, it is wise to start with conservative treatment and only progress to more-invasive options when less-invasive approaches have failed. Pain management often requires a multidisciplinary approach to address other problems that accompany the primary underlying condition and achieve an optimal result. Your pain management physician may ask you to participate in other treatments as directed by physicians in other specialties to complement the pain management treatments you are undergoing. Some practices will have all this care under one roof, and others work collaboratively with other physicians or practices in the area to accomplish the goal of comprehensive treatment. This may include elements such as medication management, physical therapy, massage, **acupuncture**, chiropractic or osteopathic manipulation, and **behavioral counseling**. These treatments are meant to help treat your pain and to get you back to living as normal a life as possible. Remember that every little bit can help.

### Physical Therapy

By the time you read this book, you may have already tried physical therapy (PT) for many weeks, perhaps months, and maybe even years. Physical therapy is an important adjunct to many of the treatments that interventional pain physicians perform. Patients are often referred for pain management evaluations when the benefits from physical therapy or chiropractic care have plateaued. Further physical therapy may be appropriate after the pain physician has alleviated some of your painful symptoms and improved your function to the point where you can again make progress with PT. Sometimes physical therapy is instituted too early: the first time you tried PT, you may have been in so much pain that you weren't able to do the exercises properly or consistently enough to benefit. More functional gains can be made when your pain is better managed.

Many excellent books are solely dedicated to physical therapy. For the purposes of this book, it's important for you to understand that your physician will likely have you involved with physical therapy and exercise before, during, and/or after your therapeutic interventions. The goals of the physical therapy program designed for you will vary from person to person. For most people, improving muscular strength is important to improve the long-term stability of the affected area. Other goals may include increased flexibility or developing proper lifting techniques and other life skills to prevent re-injury. Therapy programs are often prescribed for a specific amount of time (i.e., twice a week for six weeks), and when the program ends, patients are usually expected to continue doing the exercises on their own.

When you're injured or when a **chronic pain** condition progresses, you will often baby the area. Consider what happens when you cut your hand while cooking. For a while, you will try to avoid doing things with that hand. Once the cut heals, you return to using your hand as you did before it was injured. Now imagine that you couldn't use that hand for months or even years. Eventually you would lose strength in your hand and arm because you haven't been lifting, turning, or moving anything with that hand. Physical therapy will help you regain strength in the injured area, improve stability, and ensure proper alignment so you can return to normal activities of daily living. Treatments in which the disc is repaired (see chapter 17 on minimally invasive disc surgery) often require extensive postoperative physical therapy to stabilize and improve the function of the operative region. Physical therapy is also usually prescribed to help you regain strength and increase your ability to function following open lumbar surgeries such as microdiscectomies, fusions, or disc replacements. Physical therapy is typically used throughout the treatment of CRPS, but those who have severe dysfunction may require very lengthy courses of physical therapy to regain maximal function. These are just a few examples of how physical therapy is used to help chronic pain patients.

## Behavioral Counseling

Don't be alarmed or concerned if your physician recommends psychological evaluation, testing, or counseling; this is part of the global approach to improve your symptoms. It doesn't mean your doctor thinks you're crazy. Unfortunately, patients with chronic pain often develop secondary psychological dysfunction including depression, anxiety, and other problems. Much like physical therapy, behavioral modification and psychiatric care exist to help you deal with your chronic pain. It is also not uncommon for patients with personality disorders, pre-existing anxiety, or pre-existing depression to develop chronic pain. To effectively treat chronic pain, it is often necessary to also address underlying, and sometimes pre-existing, psychological issues that are going on simultaneously. Uncontrolled depression and anxiety can reduce the beneficial effects of other therapeutic interventions, and some insurance carriers won't cover some therapies (such as implantable techniques) if the patient has psychological issues that aren't well controlled. Mental health concerns must be addressed to optimize your long-term outcome. Again, this book is not meant to be a primer on psychological conditions or even the psychological aspects of pain, but we merely want to point out that it's often an important component of treatment in the chronic pain patient.

## Other Therapies

Other adjuvant therapies can include **TENS units**, acupuncture, chiropractic treatment, **orthotics** (shoe inserts), weight loss programs, smoking cessation, **spinal decompression therapy**, and many other treatment modalities that your interventional pain management physician may deem appropriate for your specific condition.

# CHAPTER 7

## MEDICATIONS: SO MUCH MORE THAN JUST PAIN PILLS

A variety of medications can be useful in pain treatment. This chapter will provide a brief overview of the various types of medications that are used in the treatment of **chronic pain**. As you will see, there is more to taking pain medication than popping a pill to feel better. It is extremely important to take your medications as prescribed. If your doctor sends you for blood work, remember that it's important, so don't put it off. You must also inform your doctor of all side effects you experience. What may seem embarrassing and unrelated (like constipation or sexual dysfunction) can have severe consequences. Maintain an open dialogue with your doctor about how your medications are working. The earlier side effects are reported, the better your chance of decreasing their negative effects.

## Opioids (Narcotics)

When people think of pain medications, they usually think of opioids or narcotics. Although the terms are relatively interchangeable, an opioid is a medical term used to describe medicines that work at the receptors in the brain where opium and morphine work, whereas narcotic is a legal term that describes substances with the potential for illegal use.

Opioids can be classified by their length of action. **Short-acting opioids** usually last for two to four hours and are best used for acute pain, such as the pain immediately following a broken bone or extracted tooth. Unfortunately, most pain patients have pain that lasts for hours, days, weeks, or even years, and the short-acting medicines may not be the best choice for these patients. Imagine that you were in a room with a strong smell. After a while, you would get used to the smell and you wouldn't notice it as much. But if you were to walk out of the room and then come back a few minutes later, the smell would seem much stronger than it had originally. We think the same is true with pain: if you take a short-acting pain medicine to relieve pain and then the medicine wears off, the pain may seem to return stronger than it was before you took the pain medication. We also think the "pop a pill, feel better" relief of short-acting medicines is part of what leads to addiction. So instead, we often turn to **long-acting opioids** for patients who suffer chronic pain. These forms of medication provide a sustained, steady release of medication for eight to 72 hours, depending on the delivery system used. In theory, long-acting opioids are supposed to be less addictive because they don't reinforce the behavior of popping pills. While there may be some validity to that statement, we have learned the hard way with medicines like Oxycontin® that these drugs clearly are just as addictive and perhaps more so.

Another method of classification is to divide opioids into classes based on how they are made. Medications that are directly made from opium are naturally-occurring opioids, such as morphine and codeine. Opioids that are created in the laboratory from those naturally-occurring compounds are called semisynthetic opioids, such as oxycodone and hydrocodone. **Synthetic opioids** are compounds that originated in the laboratory, such as fentanyl and methadone.

A third method of classification deals with how the opioids function. They can work by stimulating a receptor in the brain where morphine works; these pain medicines are called opioid **agonists** and include morphine as well as oxycodone, hydrocodone, fentanyl, oxymorphone, hydromorphone, and methadone. Another type of opioid is called an agonist/antagonist opioid because it antagonizes (inhibits or blocks) the receptor where morphine works and instead stimulates a different opioid receptor. Examples of agonist/**antagonist** opioids include Stadol® or Nubain®. These medicines should not be used with standard opioids because they can suddenly make those pain medicines stop working, leading to withdrawal symptoms. Pure opioid antagonists such as Narcan® are used to reverse the respiratory depressant effects of opioids.

All opioid medicines work by dulling the brain. They don't make the pain go away; it is like stuffing cotton in your ears so you don't hear the noise as much. There are several serious concerns about using opioids to treat chronic pain. Pain is often a protective mechanism that warns you of injury, so by dulling the pain response, pain medicines can potentially set up the possibility for further injury. For many chronic pain patients, however, pain has lost its protective role. Pain medicines also tend to be sedating, so patients do less rather than more, which leads to increased debilitation and deconditioning. For example, if you used to be able to run marathons and you fell and broke your leg, you wouldn't be able to run a marathon the day you get out of your cast. To get back to the level of stamina you once had, you will need to recondition your body. At first, you may need medication to perform simple activities, but your leg will eventually return to the condition it was in before you broke it, and you'll be able to stop taking the medication and return to a normal life. Pain medicines should be used to improve function and allow rehabilitation, not to get high.

## Side Effects and Complications

Because pain medicines can dull the brain, they may make you less responsive to everything around you, which may potentially make it dangerous to drive a car or operate heavy machinery. This is true of many medications but is especially true of opioids. Every individual is different; some patients do not experience these cognitive changes and can lead normal lives, including operating a car while taking pain medications. Some cannot; if you think your medications are affecting your ability to perform normal functions, you should call your doctor to discuss this right away.

People breathe less deeply and more slowly when they are taking opioids; when this is to a degree that it is dangerous, it is called **respiratory depression**. The risk of this can be increased by many factors, especially if pain medicines are mixed with other substances that cause respiratory depression (such as alcohol or tranquilizers). If left unrecognized, this can lead to coma and death. Pain medicines can also lead to poor judgment and decreased mental acuity. Patients often complain that pain medications make them feel "stupid."

Over time, pain medicines tend to become less effective, so you will require larger doses to get the same effect. This is called developing a tolerance. Tolerance occurs because the receptors in the brain become less sensitive to a medicine that is used over a long period of time. This is similar to tasting salty food. Initially, the food tastes salty, but you become accustomed to that taste over time; then food without salt tastes bland because your taste buds have become accustomed to saltiness. Some patients can be maintained on the same dosage for many years without any attenuation of effect, others have bigger problems with tolerance. The answer is, however, not to just keep increasing the medication and chasing the pain; this approach rarely works. Rotating medications, drug holidays (when no meds are taken for a period of time), and treating the underlying condition are all viable options. Sometimes just treatment of an exacerbation with an injection can bring the pain back under control and make the same medications effective again.

Physical dependence is another concern. Once your body gets used to pain medicines, you can experience withdrawal when you don't have the medicines. The more pain medicine you take, the more likely it is that your body will develop dependence. Physical dependence, however, is not necessarily the same as addiction. For example, if you are diabetic and stopped taking your **insulin**, your blood sugars would go out of control and you would get very sick. That doesn't mean you're addicted to insulin; it means that you have developed a physical need for the medicine. Addiction, on the other hand, is a drug-seeking behavior. It's a compulsive need to take the medicine despite the knowledge of its potential harm. Some people are more at risk for addiction because of a prior addiction to other substances (such as alcohol or nicotine), a family history of addiction, a history of psychological or sexual abuse, or simply being young and inexperienced with taking these medicines. Almost 10 % of the population has a gene that predisposes them to the risk of addiction. You should expect your prescribing physician to monitor you closely and intervene if they think you are becoming addicted to your medications.

Because there are also opioid receptors in the gut, taking opioids slows down the movement of the gut, so all opioids can cause constipation. Usually this is a relatively mild problem and can be easily managed with increased fluids, laxatives, and medicines to stimulate gut movement. However, if untreated, the stool can harden and you may become impacted (unable to have a bowel movement). In its most severe form, the bowel can potentially even rupture, causing widespread infection in the belly **(peritonitis)** and even death. As embarrassing as it may be, if you develop constipation from your medications, it is important that you report this to your doctors before a minor inconvenience becomes a major problem.

All opioids can release **histamine**, a compound the body makes that causes itching, welts, and swelling. Some opioids (such as morphine) tend to release more histamine than others; this does not represent an allergic reaction and actually usually gets better over time, unlike allergic reactions, which would be expected to get worse with each dosage. Opioids can cause sweating, which is usually mild but may be severe at times. Opioids also can stimulate areas in the brain, which cause nausea and vomiting. Long-term use can decrease the body's production of hormones such as estrogen and testosterone, necessitating some form of external supplementation. Hypogonadism (low hormonal levels) is becoming a much more commonly recognized complication of chronic opioids. Symptoms include fatigue, decreased sexual drive, poor pain relief, and depression.

As you can see, opioids are useful medicines to treat pain, but they also have significant and potentially severe side effects that may limit their long-term use. All side effects should be reported to your physician, who will help guide you to properly respond.

## Medication/Narcotic/Opioid Agreements and Drug Testing

Many of the medications discussed in our review have the potential for misuse, abuse, and diversion. Pain physicians commonly employ some form of patient monitoring to ensure that patients are taking their medications as prescribed and are not taking medications unknown to the doctor, whether legal or illegal.

It is important that your physician monitor the effects of any medications you are given. In the same way that some medications can cause liver or kidney damage and must be monitored closely to identify problems early, before the changes are permanent or life threatening, opioids must be monitored closely to look for early signs of addiction. Addiction can strike anyone, regardless of socioeconomic class or ethnicity, so everyone must be monitored. Because these medications have a "street value" and some people will sell or trade their medicines, your doctor will likely have you sign a treatment agreement with a series of rules that you must obey in order to continue receiving these medications. He or she will also likely periodically monitor your use of the medicines through at least one of the following methods:

1. *Urine drug testing (UDT).* Like monitoring blood sugars for a patient with diabetes on insulin, a UDT monitors the opioids in your blood stream (and therefore in the urine). Your doctor will look for the medication(s) that were prescribed, but also for

medicine(s) that were not prescribed, and for illegal drugs such as heroin or cocaine.

2. *Pill counts.* Your doctor might ask you to bring in your pill bottle to count the number of pills left to ensure you aren't taking more than was prescribed.

3. *Prescription drug monitoring programs (PDMP).* Many states monitor opioid prescriptions to identify patients who are getting pain pills from multiple doctors, almost always a sign that a patient is in trouble with their medications. At the time of this writing, 43 states have laws that have helped to establish, or that will establish, such monitoring programs. We expect that all 50 states will have such programs in the near future and that eventually this information will be shared between the various states to allow your physician to monitor medication use across state lines.

## Anti-Inflammatories

Pain is caused by inflammation. When cell membranes are damaged (for instance, by a knife blade or a bruise), they release chemicals that are metabolized into compounds called prostaglandins. Prostaglandins trigger a pain response (causing you to hold that part of your body still), increased blood flow (to bring in repair cells), and swelling. Pain from tissue trauma, infections, and irritation is caused by inflammation. Inflammation is the body's natural response to tissue injury and is helpful as a warning that this is occurring. However, once the problem is known, continuing inflammation becomes counterproductive. It can be diminished by the use of powerful drugs that inhibit the response. The two types of anti-inflammatory medications are steroid or non-steroidal anti-inflammatory agents.

## Steroids

Steroids are the strongest **anti-inflammatory medicines** available. Steroids are classified by their function. **Glucocorticosteroids** control inflammation, while **mineralocorticoid steroids** control the volume of fluid in your blood vessels and therefore blood pressure, and **androgenic steroids** are used to bulk up muscles. Your body makes steroids all the time. Steroids are produced in the body by the adrenal glands that sit on top of the kidneys, and the adrenal glands constantly measure the amount of steroid in the blood to decide how much more to make. Steroids control a wide variety of functions in your body, including the amount of sugar in your blood, the amount of calcium in your bones, the texture of your skin, the texture of your hair, the distribution of fat, the distribution of muscle, and the body's response to inflammation. In fact, steroids keep you from turning into one big blister every day, since every activity you do can create inflammation. Steroids can be used on the skin (topically), by mouth, by vein, by injection in the muscle, or in a time-release formulation injected right where the problem is located. In other chapters, you will learn about steroids placed on nerves, tendons, joints, and in the spinal column for the treatment of pain.

Steroids by mouth or by muscle injection are useful for aggressive short-term pain treatments, but they are not usually used for long-term pain management because of the potential for severe side effects. (One exception is the patient with severe chronic arthritis who may be placed on a long-term steroid regimen to treat and limit the progression of the disease.)

## Side Effects and Complications

Steroids carry the risk of multiple potential complications, and the probability of having complications depends on how much steroid actually gets into the bloodstream. The adrenal glands cannot tell the difference between each of the different types of steroids, and if the adrenals detect enough steroid and for a long enough period of time, they will cut back or potentially shut down production of the body's natural steroids. When used over long periods of time, steroids can cause elevated blood sugar and therefore diabetes, high blood pressure, osteoporosis (a lack of calcium in the bones), thinning of the skin, and changes to the distribution of fat around the shoulders (otherwise known as a dowager's hump). Most importantly, if the adrenal glands shut down, they don't make **adrenaline**, and that can be life threatening because your body needs adrenaline to help your heart beat stronger during emergencies. The classic example we see is an athlete who takes steroids to bulk up muscles (a different type of steroid than is used for pain), but remember, the body can't tell the difference between the types of steroids and the adrenal glands will start to shut down. That's fine, as long as they continue to use the steroids, but if they stop taking the steroids (so they won't test positive on a urine test, for example) and then need adrenaline to work while on the field or court, they could have a life-threatening collapse of basic body functions. Androgenic steroids can also affect the heart and lead to arrhythmias (irregular heartbeats) or a heart attack.

## Non-Steroidal Anti-Inflammatories

Interventional pain physicians also use non-steroidal **anti-inflammatories** (NSAIDs). The first of these developed was aspirin (acetylsalicyclic acid), and it is still a very effective anti-inflammatory medicine. Motrin® (ibuprofen) was introduced in 1974, and was released as an over-the-counter (OTC) medication in 1984. This was followed by Aleve® (naproxen), Feldene® (piroxicam), Lodine® (etodolac), Voltaren® (diclofenac), Oravail® (ketoprofen), and Toradol® (ketorolac), as well as many others. Today, there are too many different NSAIDs to provide a comprehensive picture of each one. This class of medications acts to reduce inflammation and swelling, thereby decreasing pain. When one doesn't work it is worth trying another, as it is often hard to predict which NSAID will work for which patient. These medicines, though not as strong as steroids, can be very effective anti-inflammatory agents, without the potential diabetes, osteoporosis, and adrenal effects.

### Side Effects and Complications

Aspirin and other NSAIDs can cause stomach ulceration and stomach bleeding, which kills 16,000 people per year. Aspirin will also prevent the platelets (small particles in the blood that help the blood to clot) from working for the life of the platelet, which is about ten days. So if you had surgery or injections done within about ten days of taking a regular dose of aspirin, you could be at an increased risk for bleeding. This is why most people are told to stop aspirin two weeks before surgery or any major invasive injections. Baby aspirin (81 mg or less) does not seem to cause as much of a platelet problem, but it is still important to check with your doctor prior to any injections. Your doctor will counsel you regarding whether or not you need to stop aspirin and for how long. Other NSAIDs inhibit the platelets for only about a day or two, and therefore have less risk of bleeding, though they still can cause significant stomach irritation and stomach bleeding.

Non-steroidal anti-inflammatory medicines can also damage the kidneys if they are taken in large doses for long periods of time. Unfortunately, because many are now available without a prescription, and, because people believe that a medication must be safe if you can buy it over the counter, a significant number of patients die because their use of these anti-inflammatory medications is not being monitored.

**Not-So-New Advances**

Around 2001, a brand new type of anti-inflammatory medicine was developed, which isolated some of the beneficial effects while limiting the negative effects. Two types of enzymes, COX 1 and COX 2, are involved in the body's response to trauma. COX 1 enzymes control the activity of the platelets and make up the protective lining of the stomach; COX 2 is involved with pain, fever, and inflammation. This new type of anti-inflammatory inhibits COX 2 (preventing pain) but not COX 1 (so there is not a problem with the platelets or the lining of the stomach). The first drug developed was celecoxib (Celebrex®) and then a second drug, rofecoxib (Vioxx®), was developed. Although these two medicines are in the same class, rofecoxib is metabolized to a medicine that interferes with the body's blood-pressure system and therefore could cause increased blood pressure (which we now know leads to an increased risk of heart attacks and strokes). Because Vioxx® was associated with a theoretical increased risk of heart attacks and strokes, it was taken off the market. Celebrex® is not metabolized in that way, does not interfere with blood pressure, and does not increase the risk of heart attacks and strokes (or at least not any more than all anti-inflammatory medications do). Celebrex®, therefore, is still on the market and may be very useful for pain immediately before and after surgery or to prevent pain from surgery. Because it doesn't cause platelet problems, Celebrex® can be used safely during surgery without an increased risk of bleeding.

## Anticonvulsants

There are several different types of pain, and each seems to respond better to particular types of medication. Nerve pain, for instance, does not respond well to opioids (except perhaps methadone). However, nerve pain responds much better to **anti-seizure medications**, also known as **anticonvulsants**. Anticonvulsants stabilize nerve membranes and prevent excessive firing of nerves that cause seizures. In a similar way, these drugs help to decrease the spontaneous firing of nerves that can be seen with nerve injuries. Anticonvulsants diminish pain by making it less likely that nerves will fire at all and lessen the intensity of the discharge when they do. Gabapentin (Neurontin®) is a drug that was initially approved by the FDA to treat seizures in children, but was later approved to treat nerve pain, once its usefulness for this indication was established.

## Side Effects and Complications

Older anti-seizure medicines, such as Dilantin® and Tegretol®, can cause significant liver and blood problems. Patients on these medications need regular blood tests to monitor liver function. Newer anti-seizure medicines such as Neurontin® (gabapentin), Topamax® (topiramate), and Lyrica® (pregabalin) do not have those same toxicities and do not need to be monitored with blood tests. All these medicines have potential for sleepiness and sedation, so they are usually started just at night. However, to get adequate pain relief, they usually need to be used in higher doses throughout the day. Your doctor will provide you with a specific schedule that will slowly get you to the dosage you need for optimal relief. You will need to use caution at first while driving or using heavy machinery because, even though these are not opioids, they can still alter your ability to function normally. Once you are on a stable dose and if you have no side effects, then it should be safe to operate a car. In general, a good rule of thumb is to try to avoid driving for 48 hours after any potentially sedating medication is started or your dosage is increased.

## Antidepressants

Patients who suffer from chronic pain have a very high rate of depression, and people who are depressed often develop chronic pain. In fact, pain treatment is rarely successful if a patient is experiencing depression that isn't being adequately treated. **Antidepressants** are an extremely important tool in the management of pain. Several different classes of medications have antidepressant qualities:

### Tricyclic Antidepressants (TCAs)

These medicines (such as amitriptyline, desipramine, and trazodone) are some of the earliest antidepressants and can be very effective for treating some types of nerve pain such as peripheral neuropathy, migraines, and fibromyalgia. Unfortunately, they also have a variety of side effects including dry mouth, constipation, irregular heartbeat, and a drop in blood pressure when you stand up. Trazodone can increase the risk of prolonged erection (priapism) in males, which can lead to impotence if untreated. On the other hand, the sedative property of tricyclics can be useful in treating insomnia, and these medications are usually used at nighttime in low doses (much lower doses than when used to treat depression). Of all the antidepressants, tricyclic antidepressants have the most evidence of working well, and they are still often used as first-line drugs in pain management.

### Selective Serotonin Reuptake Inhibitors (SSRIs)

Serotonin is one of the major chemicals in the brain, and a lack of serotonin is associated with depression. Selective serotonin reuptake inhibitors (SSRIs) prevent the body from breaking down serotonin and therefore raise the serotonin levels at the nerve endings. Prozac® (fluoxetine) was the first SSRI developed, and there are now several others, such as Zoloft® (sertraline), Paxil® (paroxetine), Celexa® (citalopram), and Lexapro® (escitalopram). Although these medicines are very effective for treating depression and have fewer side effects than tricyclic antidepressants, there is no good evidence of their usefulness in treating painful conditions, unless the pain is being caused by depression itself. These medications can potentially cause a significant decrease in sexual drive and/or pleasure, which could potentially lead to marital unhappiness.

### Serotonin Norepinephrine Reuptake Inhibitors (SNRIs)

Another chemical in the brain involved with depression is norepinephrine (noradrenaline). This compound is similar to adrenaline (also known as epinephrine), which is produced by the adrenal glands, but norepinephrine is made in the brain. Serotonin norepinephrine reuptake inhibitor (SNRI) medications prevent the body from breaking down norepinephrine and serotonin, which allows both levels to increase in the brain and reverse depression. Medications such as Effexor® (venlafaxine) and Cymbalta® (duloxetine) fall into this category. These seem to have fewer sexual side effects, and good evidence exists to show they are effective for pain relief. In fact, Cymbalta® is approved by the FDA for treatment of both depression and painful diabetic peripheral neuropathy. Because of the increase of norepinephrine, SNRIs may be associated with elevated blood pressure and agitation.

## Anti-Anxiety Medications (Anxiolytics)

Many chronic pain patients also feel as though they have anxiety. Depression is also often misdiagnosed as anxiety. But many patients do not realize that adrenaline (epinephrine), which is released by the body when it is under stress, will cause symptoms of anxiety such as a rapid heart rate, agitation, nervousness, and difficulty sleeping. Unfortunately, **anxiolytic** medicines such as Valium® (diazepam) or Xanax® (alprazolam) only mask the symptoms and are also potentially addictive. These medicines work at the same level of the brain as alcohol and, just like with alcohol, the feeling of relief is only an illusion. Most of us realize that using alcohol to "steady nerves" or to "relax" or to "get through the day" are signs of alcohol dependence; yet we have patients using those same words to describe the need for **anti-anxiety medications**. If you are having symptoms of anxiety, it is important to identify why you have the symptoms and to treat the cause of the anxiety, not the symptoms. Most pain doctors avoid these kinds of medicines for long-term use because of the potential for addiction.

## Muscle Relaxants

When a body part is injured, the muscles around that area go into spasm to protect the injured structure by limiting movement. Unfortunately, this decreased movement can actually cause more pain, and a decrease in mobility leads to deconditioning and a downward spiral in function. Therefore, muscle relaxants are used to prevent this part of the body's natural response mechanism. Most muscle relaxers, such as Skelaxin®, Robaxin®, and Flexeril®, only work indirectly on the skeletal muscles themselves. Instead, most muscle relaxants work in the brain to decrease the number of spasm signals, so they only work indirectly on the muscles. This is also the way that medicines like Valium® (diazepam) and Soma® (carisoprodol) work. Though frequently prescribed, Soma® can be a dangerous compound because it is metabolized to a very addictive medicine that has been taken off the market. Soma®, like alcohol, increases the risk of respiratory depression and death from opioids, and should not be a first-line muscle relaxant. Pain physicians sometimes use more powerful muscle relaxants such as baclofen and Zanaflex® (tizanidine), which were originally used to treat spasticity of spinal cord injuries and cerebral palsy. Unlike Valium® and Soma®, **baclofen** and Zanaflex® are not addictive and actually treat the muscle spasticity itself. Prolonged muscle spasm is usually related to an underlying cause that, if treatable, should be addressed rather than trying to treat spasm that has an underlying stimulus. For instance, chronic spasm on one side of the back can be due to a leg length discrepancy, which causes an altered gait. A shoe lift may resolve the problem. Alternatively, the spasm could be secondary to a **disc herniation** and require treatment directed at this problem.

## Medical Marijuana

Very few medications are as controversial as marijuana. It has been used as a medicine for thousands of years, but the FDA considers it a highly abusable drug with no legitimate medical purpose. Under federal law, it is a controlled, illegal substance. To make matters more confusing, 14 states have defied the federal government and made **medical marijuana** legal. The federal government has not decided what to do at this point, but to date there has been no major show down over these conflicting laws. Pain physicians have to grapple with this inconsistency when deciding how to deal with the patient who is using marijuana.

Marijuana contains cannabinoids, chemical compounds named after the plant's genus, *Cannabis*. Cannabinoid receptors are found throughout the body: in the brain, in the gut, in the eyes, and on white blood cells. The presence of cannabinoid receptors and the known positive effects that it causes would suggest that there is some role for medical marijuana. It has been touted to help glaucoma, **chemotherapy**-induced nausea, and medical-related weight loss (for example, from cancer or HIV). Research in this area is growing but is slow to arrive. Perhaps this is because most research money comes from federal government funding and since they consider it illegal, it has been hard to conduct research that would determine just what these compounds actually do and, therefore, define the role of medical marijuana.

Even if it does have a medicinal role, unscrupulous doctors have been prescribing medical marijuana to anyone who has the cash to pay for it, and "pot mills" have sprung up all over the country. In California, it has been estimated that there are more medical marijuana clinics than there are McDonald's restaurants. Until more research is done, most legitimate pain doctors will be very leery of medical marijuana and will prescribe it very sparingly, if at all, to carefully selected patients.

# CHAPTER 8

# TRIGGER POINT INJECTIONS: TREATING TIGHT AND RESTRICTED MUSCLES

Muscles are actually made of millions of microscopic muscle fibers that consist of two proteins that come together and interlock, like the fingers of your hands. Muscles require oxygen and nutrients to contract and release. When they don't get the oxygen that they need to release them from the contracted state, they can end up in a state of spasm. Trigger points occur when over-stimulated muscle fibers do not have enough oxygen to release from their interlocked state. Trigger point pain, also called myofascial pain, describes a condition in muscles that results from a lack of blood flow (ischemia) in a section of muscle: tiny contractions, or knots, develop in a muscle when it is injured or overworked. Trigger points affect muscles by keeping them both tight (because of the spasm) and weak (because the muscle is chronically overworked). These taut bands of muscle keep constant tension on the muscle's attachments, which causes inflammation of the tendon (**tendonitis**), and tension on the joint capsule, which causes joint pain (**arthralgia**). The constant tension in the fibers of the trigger point itself restricts blood flow in the immediate muscle region; this causes an accumulation of metabolic byproducts such as lactic acid, which cause soreness in the muscle and stimulates more spasm, creating a vicious cycle.

Those resulting knots or taut bands in the muscles can cause local pain. This is often misdiagnosed as arthritis. The knots are very irritable, and pressure on them (or touching the spot with a needle) can cause the muscle to twitch or jump. They may also cause pain in other areas of the body, a phenomenon called **referred pain**. This can result in headaches, neck and jaw pain, hand pain, abdominal pain, pelvic pain, and foot and leg pain. Trigger points can also mimic heartburn, heart attacks, appendicitis, migraines, and **sciatica** as well as cause dizziness, nausea, heart **arrhythmias**, and numbness of the hands and feet. When some muscles develop trigger points, the spasm or contracture of that musculature can place pressure on adjacent nervous structures and mimic pain from nerve compression, causing pain going down the leg or arm (**pseudoradicular symptoms**) (figure 8.1).

Because the symptoms can be so diverse, and because the pain may be coming from an area widely separated from the muscle that is causing the pain, the origin of myofascial pain can often be difficult to pinpoint. This diagnostic dilemma is exemplified by the experience some people have during a heart attack in which they have arm pain but don't have chest pain. That pain pattern occurs because the nerves that go to the heart and the nerves that go to the arm come together at the same level of the spinal column, and the brain interprets the pain as coming from the arm. If doctors didn't recognize that pain pattern, patients might be sent for arm x-rays instead of an EKG to evaluate the heart.

Recognizing the pattern of pain when taking a history and identifying the painful points that can be felt on physical exam can give the pain physician clues to the cause of the pain. Unfortunately, trigger point pain referral patterns are not always recognized, and there is no equivalent of an EKG for diagnosis of the problem. Most conventional approaches to the treatment of pain generally operate on the assumption that the cause of pain will be found at the site of the pain. Trigger points almost always cause pain elsewhere, and although the trigger point site might be painful as well, sometimes there is only pain at the referral site, like in the heart attack/arm example. The best way to confirm the diagnosis is by injecting local anesthetic into the affected muscle to see if the pain goes away.

Activation of trigger points may be caused by a number of factors. These may include acute or chronic muscle overload, activation by other trigger points, or disorders such as an underactive thyroid. Psychological distress, chemical imbalances such as low potassium, hormone imbalances such as low estrogen, direct trauma to the region, nerve irritation, infections, and health issues such as smoking can also cause trigger points.

Fibromyalgia is another condition that is often mistaken for trigger point pain. Fibromyalgia is characterized by widespread pain and tenderness and is thought to be related to increased brain recognition of pain that gives rise to deep tissue tenderness that includes muscles. Trigger point or myofascial pain is pain from muscles and fascia (the lining of the muscles). These two distinct problems must be correctly identified to be effectively treated. Physicians who specialize in fibromyalgia usually manage the diagnosis and treatment of fibromyalgia, and it is beyond the scope of this book.

Trigger points can be secondary to other underlying injuries/problems and may accompany many other painful conditions, representing another component of the **chronic pain** syndrome. Treatment of the primary underlying problem often leads to spontaneous resolution of the associated secondary trigger points. If symptoms don't improve with treatment directed solely at a **myofascial pain syndrome**, then one should look for other underlying conditions that may be causing the secondary trigger points to occur.

## Treatment Options

A common treatment for trigger point pain involves injections given in the office. These injections (often simply called trigger point injections) may be classified as "active" or "latent" (present, but not active) and also as "key" (primary) versus "satellite" (secondary). Sometimes there are trigger points present that aren't causing you current pain symptoms. Primary trigger points are the ones causing the majority of your symptoms, and secondary ones, while painful, are not the primary cause of your pain. Successfully treating the key trigger point will often resolve the satellite trigger points, but occasionally the satellites need treatment too or they stimulate the other triggers to recur.

Injections provide immediate relief and can confirm the diagnosis. If injection of a trigger point in the back relieves chest pain, you can be pretty certain that the chest pain is not related to your heart. These injections into muscles should be of local anesthetic only, because steroids in the muscles can cause tissue damage. This does not totally negate the use of steroids, because it may be reasonable to inject steroids into inflamed tendons. **Dry needling** (placing needles into specific points of the muscle without injecting medicine) can be just as effective but may cause more post-injection soreness. **Botulinum toxin** (more widely recognized as Botox®) may occasionally be indicated, if trigger point injections give only temporary relief. Botox® can provide more sustained relief; however, it can be difficult to get approval from your insurance carrier because the drug is more widely recognized for its cosmetic uses. Botox® injections cannot be injected into the same muscle group more often than once every three months. Sarapin® (the extract of the pitcher plant) has also been used to provide more sustained relief.

Doctors and physical therapists may use deep tissue massage (neuromuscular therapy), pulsed **ultrasound**, **electrostimulation**, **ischemic compression (acupressure)**, dry needling, "spray and stretch" using a cooling (vapo-coolant) spray, or low-level laser therapy in place of, or in conjunction with, injections. In addition to formal physical therapy, it is extremely important that the patient perform a stretching program at home between physical therapy sessions. A successful treatment protocol relies on identifying trigger points, deactivating the trigger points, and then stretching the affected muscles along their natural range of motion and length. If the stretching is not performed, the muscle will simply return to its original position where trigger points are likely to redevelop.

# CHAPTER 9

## PERIPHERAL NERVE BLOCKS: INJECTIONS IN OTHER PLACES AND SPACES

Your body is covered with nerves, both on the skin and in the deep tissues. Central nerves are those in the spinal column and brain; **peripheral nerves** are those outside the spinal column. Each of these nerves goes to a different part of the body, and when these nerves are trapped, they cause pain in a predictable pattern. Nerves travel in pathways and canals, and swelling can trap them. You can visualize those nerves as your finger, and the canal they run in would be a ring on that finger. If your finger is traumatized and starts to swell, it becomes hard to pull off the ring—and the harder you try to pull off the ring, the more swollen the finger becomes.

Nerve entrapment can also cause pain in areas of the body other than the site of entrapment. This is called **"referred pain."** As an example, when someone is having a heart attack, he may feel pain going down his arm but may not have any chest pain at all. This is because the nerves that go to the heart come into the spinal column at the same level as the arm nerves, and the brain interprets that pain as coming from the arm. Without knowing this referral pattern, a physician might mistakenly think the problem is coming from the nerves in the neck and recommend surgery instead of an evaluation by a **cardiologist.**

An injection by an interventional pain physician can numb a nerve, and, if that makes the pain go away, it confirms the cause of the pain. At the same time, the pain physician can add a time-released steroid medication, which acts to decrease swelling. Peripheral nerve blocks, then, can be both diagnostic and therapeutic; in other words, these injections can help make the diagnosis as well as treat the problem. In this chapter we will discuss some of the most common nerve entrapments, although many others are now recognized.

As you will see, peripheral nerve entrapments can occur from the top of the head to the toes. A knowledgeable interventional pain physician can diagnose the issue and treat the nerves in an effective manner. Knowing the cause of pain can help the physician treat the problem effectively and will decrease unnecessary and potentially dangerous surgeries and therapies.

## Head and Neck

The **supraorbital nerve** runs from the top of the eye to the forehead (figure 9.1). This nerve can become trapped by frowning, squinting, and fluid retention (such as just before a woman's menstrual period). This is often mistaken for migraines, sinusitis, and cluster headaches.

The **infraorbital nerve** comes out of the skull just below the eye and sends branches to the upper teeth (figure 9.1). Blows to the face, cheek fractures, or dental procedures can injure this nerve, and smiling or brushing your teeth can irritate the nerve. Patients often have multiple dental procedures or are misdiagnosed as having sinusitis when this nerve is inflamed.

The **mental nerve** is found near the point of the chin, and it gives sensation to the lower lip and teeth (figure 9.1). This nerve can be injured during dental procedures and by jaw trauma or dentures.

The **auriculotemporal nerve** is the nerve most commonly associated with headaches and migraines (figure 9.1). Located in the temple next to an artery, this nerve can be irritated by the muscle in the temple, especially with chewing or clenching.

The **occipital nerves** are located at the back of the head and are a common cause of migraines (figure 9.1). These nerves can be injured as they pass between the upper bones of the neck (such as is seen with whiplash) or irritated by the muscles of the shoulder and neck, which attach at the base of the skull around these nerves.

## Upper Limb

The **suprascapular nerve** runs along the top of the shoulder blade and gives sensation to the muscles of the shoulder and the shoulder joint itself. Car accidents (especially when clenching the steering wheel) or lifting objects like suitcases can cause trauma to this nerve, which causes pain to radiate down the arm and mimics a pinched nerve in the neck.

The **radial nerve** (see figure 9.2) can be trapped several places along the arm. It can be injured on the upper arm (by fractures of the upper arm bone, or **humerus**), at the elbow (referred to as **lateral epicondylitis**), or on the thumb side of the forearm (superficial radial nerve). All these will cause pain to radiate down the arm to the thumb side of the hand and can mimic pinched nerves in the neck.

In the same way, the **ulnar nerve** (figure 9.2), which goes to the little-finger side of the hand, can be trapped or traumatized at the elbow (the "funny bone") and, less commonly, at the wrist. Injection of this nerve at the level of the elbow (at the funny bone) is generally not considered safe due to the high risk of injury to the nerve with injection into a very tight canal.

The most commonly diagnosed peripheral nerve entrapment is the median nerve at the wrist. This nerve, which goes primarily to the middle finger, travels through an arch of bones in the wrist (the **carpal bones**). There is a **ligament** that goes across this C-shaped arch of bones, which then makes a canal or tunnel (figure 9.2); this entrapment is commonly called carpal tunnel syndrome, and it's usually diagnosed with a test called a **nerve conduction study.** It is important to remember, however, that not all pain going down to the hand comes from a median nerve entrapment, and in some studies, as many as 15 % of patients with no symptoms at all will have positive nerve conduction studies. **Diagnostic injections** are therefore important to confirm the diagnosis before surgery, and because these injections treat the swelling, they often can help avoid the need for surgery.

## Chest and Abdomen

**Intercostal nerves**, the nerves that travel under each rib from the spine around to the front, can be injured by rib fractures, thoracic surgery, and infections such as shingles (figure 9.3). The lower intercostal nerves actually travel around to the upper abdomen and can get trapped at the edge of the **rectus abdominus**, the muscle that runs vertically from the bottom of the breastbone to the top of the pubic bones. This muscle is what creates the "six-pack abs" on body builders. Nerves trapped at the edge of this muscle can mimic gallbladder disease or stomach ulcers.

The nerves coming out of the upper back also travel around to the front of the abdomen and can be trapped by the same muscle. These nerves, which are called the subgastric, ilioinguinal, and iliohypogastric nerves, will mimic appendicitis on the right and diverticulitis on the left, as well as endometriosis and **interstitial cystitis** (figure 9.3). Pain worsens with bearing down, coughing, bowel movement, and lifting. Women often notice increased pain with menstruation and sexual intercourse. Irritation of these nerves can result in referred pain to the testicles or vaginal area, inner thigh, or upper back.

The **genitofemoral nerve** also comes from the upper back, but it travels deep in the belly until it crosses over at the top of the pubic bone into the testicles or vaginal region. This nerve may be injured by abdominal surgery but is more commonly injured with "bikini" incisions (transverse lower abdominal) or hernia repairs. The genitofemoral nerve carries signals into the genital region as well as the inner thigh, and is often a cause of pelvic pain, especially during sexual intercourse.

The pudendal nerve gives sensation to the area between the tailbone and the pubic bone. This nerve can be traumatized by bicycle seats and straddling injuries and is unfortunately a very common cause of pain after childbirth.

## Lower Back

Turning our attention now to the back, there are several peripheral nerves that can cause pain to be felt in the back, buttock, and/ or leg. Because the term "**sciatica**" is often used interchangeably with **radiculopathy** (i.e. leg pain from a herniated disc), when leg pain is caused by something other than this, it is often called "**pseudosciatica**" or "fake sciatica" to differentiate between causes (figure 9.4). Studies have shown that as many as 30 to 60 % of patients with no back pain at all had bulging or herniated **discs** on MRI, so it's important to make the right diagnosis. Operating on a herniated disc that isn't causing pain won't make someone better.

The **cluneal nerve** comes from the top of the lower back region and travels across the top of the hip bones (the iliac crest) to send signals into the buttocks and potentially down the leg (figure 9.5). The **superior gluteal nerve** lies lower in the buttocks, above the muscle running from the tailbone to the side of the hipbone (the **piriformis muscle**) and enters the spinal column at the same level as the **sciatic nerve** (figure 9.5). This piriformis muscle can also trap the sciatic nerve and mimic a herniated disc.

## Lower Limb

The **femoral nerve** runs from the groin onto the front of the leg and then down the inner leg to the foot (figure 9.6). One of the biggest branches of the femoral nerve is the saphenous nerve. On the inner side of the knee is a small branch of the **saphenous nerve**; because it runs underneath the kneecap **(patella),** it is called the **infrapatellar saphenous nerve**. This nerve can be traumatized by knee surgery, especially **arthroscopy** or total knee replacement, and can cause generalized pain, swelling, and redness, mimicking infection. The superficial saphenous nerve travels down past the inner side of the ankle where it can be injured from out-turning ankle injuries and sprains. It can also be trapped at the big toe by bunions or tight-fitting shoes.

On the outer side of the knee is the **peroneal nerve**, a branch of the sciatic nerve. It can be traumatized at the bottom of the knee by a tight-fitting cast, which will cause weakness of the foot termed **"foot drop."** It splits into two branches. The **superficial peroneal branch** travels in front of the outer side of the ankle where it can be injured by in-turning ankle sprains or fractures of the thin bone in the lower leg called the fibula (the big bone is called the tibia). This nerve then spreads out onto the top of the foot.

Between the bones of the foot are the **digital nerves**. The digital nerve between the big toe and the second toe is the second branch of the peroneal nerve—the **deep peroneal nerve**. The others are named for the bones they lie between; for instance, the digital nerve between the fourth and fifth toes is called digital 4/5. Chronic trauma to the nerves by tight shoes can cause a mass to grow on the nerve called a **Morton's neuroma.** Though this classically occurs between the third and fourth toes, it can occur between any of the toes.

The inner side of the heel is **innervated** by the **medial calcaneal nerve,** which is often mistaken for **plantar fasciitis**. A similar nerve on the outer side is called the **lateral calcaneal nerve.** These will cause heel pain and are often associated with in-turning or out-turning of the foot with walking.

## Treatment Options

To confirm the diagnosis of a peripheral nerve injury as the cause of pain, your pain physician may recommend a peripheral nerve block. When the nerve is blocked with local anesthetic, pain caused by that nerve should typically go away. This could include all of the pain or part of the pain, depending on whether the symptoms are coming from one or more structure(s); it is not uncommon for nerve injuries to be associated with other primary or secondary musculoskeletal problems.

Once you have diagnosed a nerve as the cause of pain, how do you treat it? The diagnostic injections, which usually consist of local anesthetic and steroid (anti-inflammatory medication), often provide lasting relief. However, if the injection provides only temporary relief, there are a few longer-term options. Surgery can release the nerve, but subsequent scar tissue can re-entrap the nerve.

Nerve-killing fluids such as alcohol or **phenol** can create inflammation and scarring and should be avoided except in cancer pain or with spasticity associated with spinal cord injuries. Burning the nerve with radio frequency lesioning can also cause more inflammation and increased pain. Some physicians are using pulsed radio frequency lesioning (lower temperatures and less destruction by pulsing the energy), although the jury is still out as to the exact mechanism of action and the level of effectiveness of this approach. **Cryoneuroablation** is still likely the best option to treat these nerve entrapments (see chapter 13). A non-destructive option which is gaining some popularity is peripheral nerve stimulation (see chapter 20).

When peripheral nerves are damaged, sometimes the body responds in an exaggerated fashion, this 'wind-up' of the nervous system can result in the development of a diffuse pain syndrome, involving a much larger area of the body (usually an extremity). When this occurs it is referred to as **complex regional pain syndrome** type II or **causalgia** (see chapter 18).

# CHAPTER 10

## EPIDURAL INJECTIONS: NOT JUST FOR CHILDBIRTH

$M$ost people are familiar with epidurals as a part of childbirth. When a male patient hears that he needs an epidural to treat his back pain, a puzzled expression crosses his face. Inevitably, the next question we hear is, "Doc, isn't that what they did for my wife when she was having a baby?" Epidural steroid injections are one of the most commonly used interventional pain procedures today, and they can be used for a wide variety of different problems. There are many different types of epidural steroid injections. Epidurals for childbirth are very different from epidurals for low back pain. What makes the epidural given to the pregnant woman and the typical epidural given to the pain patient different is the type and amount of medication used in the injection, as well as the exact technique and location.

Part of the confusion about this common procedure stems from the fact that many people refer to epidurals as "blocks," but the more accurate term is "epidural steroid injection." This tells you where the injection is being done (the **epidural space**) and what is being injected (steroids). A "block" is a generic term that can apply to many different types of injections. Specifically, epidural steroid injections involve placement of steroid medication into and around the nerves of the spine to treat nerve irritation and inflammation. These injections can be performed at just about any level of the spine, although the technique may vary in location, including the cervical, thoracic, lumbar, and caudal regions.

Nerves in the spine can become irritated from a variety of causes including nerve compression, nerve trauma, stenosis (narrowing of the canal), or a herniated and/or **leaking disc. Disc herniation** is perhaps the most well-known cause of **sciatica** (from the Greek word for leg pain), that mysterious ailment that plagued our parents and grandparents. Sciatica is often unfairly relegated to the category of "old people complaints," but it can happen to anyone at any age. Sciatica is really a generic term that refers to irritation or inflammation of nerves that go to the legs. Your physician more likely will properly refer to this as a **radiculopathy** or radiculitis when the nerve irritation occurs at the level of the spine. Think about the nerves of your back as long strings that run from your spine to your legs. If you light the string on fire at the base (near your spine), eventually the fire will spread to the other end of the string (your foot) so an injured nerve in your back can cause you to feel pain in the foot if that is where the nerve ends. The site of pain doesn't tell us what caused it, so we try to avoid general terms like sciatica and instead strive to be specific to identify the cause of the pain. Some specific causes of radiculopathy include nerve compression/irritation from a herniated disc (figure 4.2) or bone build-up from arthritis (bone build-up can cause nerve compression, see figure 4.3).

If you shut your hand in a car door, it hurts; it still hurts when you take your hand out of the door, and then your hand swells. Single nerves (or nerve roots) are no different than your hand. They don't like being compressed, and the affected area can swell. Now imagine that the **spinal canal** is a ring on that swollen hand; the more the finger swells, the tighter the ring gets, and then the more the finger swells. Swelling keeps pressure on the nerves, and the nerves become irritated. This compression or nerve irritation in the spine causes you to feel pain in the area where that nerve normally registers sensation: arm nerves (cervical) cause arm pain, mid-back (thoracic) nerves cause rib pain, and leg nerves (lumbar or sacral) cause leg pain.

Nerve irritation/compression from overgrowth of bone and/or ligamentous structures is referred to as **spinal stenosis.** Stenosis refers to a narrowing of the spinal canal and can occur in the central part of the spine or off to the sides where the nerve exits the spine, also referred to as the **lateral recess** or foraminal stenosis, depending on how far out to the side the narrowing occurs.

A third cause of irritation is chemical irritation. Each disc in your back is filled with a gel-like substance that creates a cushion between the **discs**. When the cushion becomes damaged, it can crack or tear, and some of the fluid can leak out of the disc. This fluid can irritate the surrounding nerves. It is like pouring alcohol on a cut. The alcohol irritates the cut and it hurts, but when the alcohol is washed away, the burning goes away.

The key with all **interventional pain management** procedures, including epidural steroid injections, is to place the medication as close as possible to the area of injury or inflammation. When the nerve is compressed from either a disc herniation or bone overgrowth affecting the central spinal canal, then placing an epidural steroid injection in the center of the spine (also called an **interlaminar** or midline epidural steroid injection) may be an appropriate technique (figure 4.4 and 10.1 a and b). Often the location of the problem is off to the side of the spinal canal (also known as the lateral recess) or along the hole where the nerve exits the spinal column, the neuroforamen, (see chapter 4). In this case, an injection into the foramen, an area which is closer to the nerve compression, is more likely to help. When the needle is placed into the foramen, it is called a transforaminal injection (figure 10.2).

Another technique commonly employed in the lower back region is a **caudal epidural steroid injection**. In this technique, a needle is placed though an opening just above the tailbone. Dye is injected to demonstrate appropriate spread of contrast, and then medicine is injected (figure 10.3 a and b).

Using a **catheter** is another way to perform epidural steroid injections. "Catheter" is another word that people cringe at when mentioned, but your pain management doctor is not placing a catheter into your bladder. In this technique, a needle is placed into the spine and then a catheter—a thin, flexible, hollow tube—is inserted through the needle, pushed out the tip of the needle, and then steered into the area of nerve inflammation. The **injectate** (medications, such as steroids and local anesthetics) is then placed into that area and the needle and catheter are removed (figure 10.4). This is a common technique in the neck or cervical region and also in the caudal region for specific purposes, such as treating scar tissue in patients who have had prior surgery (see chapter 14).

For most types of epidurals, contrast (dye) is injected prior to the steroid to prove that the needle is in the correct location and the medication is spreading appropriately. For IPM (in contrast to labor or operative epidurals), this procedure must be performed under radiologic guidance so your doctor has a clear view of the area and can precisely document the location of the final needle position since they typically target a specific nerve or level and want to know the response at that specific site. Your doctor will inject contrast into the area, then watch as the dye appears on the picture screen of the **C-arm** (the machine that provides radiological guidance), paying particular attention to the direction in which it spreads. Some patients are concerned because of a history of contrast allergy, but the contrast that is typically used for epidural steroid injections and interventional pain management procedures has a very low risk for allergic reaction (and does not closely correlate with a CT scan or intravenous dye allergy). Except in the most extreme cases, it is usually safer to inject the contrast to accurately determine the placement of the needle (before placement of the local and steroid) than it is to perform the injection without this information.

## Possible Complications

The most common complication that can occur from an epidural steroid injection is a **"wet tap,"** or **dural puncture,** which happens when the needle punctures the membrane overlying the spinal fluid (the dura). Spinal fluid can then leak through the hole created by the needle, which can lead to a post-dural puncture headache, commonly called a spinal headache. **Postdural puncture headaches** can occur after spinal taps or lumbar punctures as well as after interventional pain procedures. The spinal fluid contained within the spine communicates with the fluid that supports the brain. The leakage of spinal fluid means there is also less spinal fluid for the brain to float in. So when you stand up, the brain sags or falls away from the skull and stretches veins that run between the surface of the brain and the skull internally, which causes a headache. Common treatments include increased oral fluids (as much as half a gallon per day), increased caffeine consumption (which causes **vasoconstriction**, or shrinking of these blood vessels), or an abdominal binder to increase the pressure in the belly, which increases the pressure of the fluid within the spinal canal and forces fluid from the spinal region back into the head. But the most effective treatment is an **epidural blood patch**. With this technique the patient's own blood is injected into the epidural space at the location of the initial needle puncture to seal the hole where the spinal fluid is leaking; this forces spinal fluid up toward the head, which provides almost immediate headache relief. Epidural blood patches have a very high effectiveness rate (greater than 95 %) and usually work almost immediately. Patients often refer to it as a "miracle cure."

Other possible complications include bleeding, infection, nerve injury or trauma, and spinal cord injury.

## After the Procedure

Patients should follow up with either the ordering physician or the doctor who performed the procedure about two weeks after the procedure to discuss the results of the injection. You may feel relief immediately after the procedure; this is likely due to the local anesthetic used in the injection, and its effects will wear off in one to three hours. The steroids used in the injection typically take three to seven days to start working and reach peak effect in ten to fourteen days (maybe a little more quickly for a transforaminal approach). This means you may not have an accurate assessment as to how well the injection worked until at least two weeks have passed. You may not notice improvement all at once, so your physician may ask you to keep a pain journal to assist in gauging the injection's effects. Patients are often better able to see a progression of relief when they keep a daily account of their symptoms. It is important to record not only pain relief but also any increase in activity or ability to function. You may not think you are better, but then all of a sudden you realize you are able to rake your yard for the first time in months. Just be aware that this increase in activity may cause soreness in muscles you haven't used in a while.

Epidural steroid injections are typically performed in a series of one to three injections. If a patient achieves 80 % or greater reduction in their symptoms with full return of function, it is not uncommon to hold off on further injections. If a patient achieves 100 % relief from the first injection, there is no indication for further injections unless symptoms recur. If an individual receives some partial benefit or pain continues to restrict his or her activity level despite a marked improvement in resting pain, a series of injections may still be indicated. It is not uncommon for patients to receive a series of two to three injections for maximal relief. These injections are typically limited to three or four in a six-month period due to the potential risks of repetitive steroid exposure (such as adrenal suppression). If the first injection doesn't help, your physician may recommend a second injection at a different level or via a different technique, or he or she may begin to look at other structures as the possible cause of your pain.

It is not uncommon for patients with complicated injuries, especially those who have undergone previous surgery, to receive intermittent, as-needed epidural injections for long-term control of their symptoms. It is also not uncommon for patients with chronic radicular (nerve root) or lower extremity pain following surgery to be maintained on medications with intermittent injections used in conjunction to control those symptoms on a long-term basis. The need for repeat injections isn't an indication that the procedure failed, but rather that the beneficial effects of the steroid have worn off. If the steroid effect is of too short a duration, then this won't be a long-term solution for the patient; if repeated injections don't provide relief for extended periods of time, then there is no indication for continued repeat injections. Some patients will come in for an epidural every six to twelve months and view it as a "tune-up." They're happy with how they feel and function well while the epidural is working, and they come back when the injection begins to wear off. These people are usually able to avoid using high-dosage, long-term medications and to avoid more invasive surgery. Only your pain management physician can provide a definitive answer as to whether or not this procedure will work for you, but it is an important option to consider.

## Questions to Ask Before Your Epidural:

1. Will this injection be performed under **fluoroscopic guidance**? As we stated earlier in the chapter, IPM procedures involving the spine should be done with radiologic guidance for safety and accuracy. **"Blind" epidural injections** (those done without x-ray guidance) have been shown to be in the wrong place more than 30 % of the time, even in experienced hands.

2. What approach or technique will you use?

3. At what level will the procedure be performed?

4. Will you use sedation? Do I need sedation?

5. Are there any restrictions after the procedure?

6. What complications can occur?

## Before the Procedure:

1. Make sure your doctor is aware of all medications you are taking. Some heart medications are **blood thinners** and will increase the risk of bleeding complications. In order to safely perform the epidural, these medications must be stopped for a certain amount of time before the procedure (at the discretion of the physician

providing you with those medications). You may also need to go for blood work the morning of the procedure to make sure your blood is clotting properly.

2. If you are diabetic, you must tell your physician ahead of time. **Insulin**-dependent diabetics will have to follow specific instructions before and after the injection. If you are having sedation during your procedure, you will need to not eat (fast) before the procedure and you should bring your insulin with you to the procedure. You may also have some variations in your blood sugar levels for up to two weeks from the steroids in the injection. If you are diabetic, it is important that you monitor your blood sugar more closely for those two weeks after the injection (or until your blood sugar is back under control). If you have a problem getting your blood sugar back into a normal range, consult the doctor managing your diabetes.

# CHAPTER 11

---

## FACET INJECTIONS: TREATING ARTHRITIS OF THE SPINE

W hen the average person hears he needs facet injections, the first question we hear is, "Where are my **facet joints**?" Everyone is familiar with the joints we can see, such as the knees, hips, and elbows, but many people don't know these very important facet joints exist. Facet joints are paired structures located between each of the vertebral bodies that act as connections between each of the spinal bones. At each spinal level, a disc separates the adjacent vertebral bones in the front of the spine; in the back of the spine, the vertebral bones are separated by these paired joints (figure 4.5).

There are many causes of axial or spinal pain, and one common cause is the **degeneration** and/or injury of the facet joints (also known as **zygapophyseal joints**). These joints can be damaged by degenerative wear-and-tear processes and/or traumatic events, both of which can cause **chronic pain** in the neck (cervical), mid-back (thoracic), or lower back (lumbar) regions. As a disc degenerates, it can place additional pressure on these joints, causing pain in this area. Traumatic injuries that strain, stretch, or tear the capsule of the joint can also cause pain in these areas.

There are seven **cervical vertebral bones,** labeled C1 to C7. There are also 12 thoracic vertebral bones labeled T1 to T12 and five **lumbar vertebral bones** labeled L1 to L5 (figure 4.1). The five tailbone vertebrae are usually fused together, except at the very tip, which is called the **coccyx.** At each spinal level, from C2–C3 at the base of the head to L5–S1 at the level of the hips, there are paired facet joints on each side of the body. Above C2–C3 there are paired joints on each side called the **atlanto-axial (AA) joints**. These joints are located between C1 and C2. The **atlanto-occipital (AO) joint** is located between the **occiput** (base of the skull) and C1 (see chapter 4 for a more detailed description of these structures). Any one of these paired joints on either or both sides can cause pain.

Certain joints refer pain, or cause pain to be experienced in very specific areas, and this is especially true in the cervical region. These common referral patterns often help physicians to determine which joints are involved in a particular pain syndrome. Injection or blockade of these joints can result in symptomatic relief. The upper cervical facet joints typically cause pain in the neck associated with headaches and pain that radiates toward the top of the shoulder. As we move lower in the neck to C5–C6 and C6–C7, pain tends to radiate between the shoulder blades (an area referred to as **periscapular**) and sometimes into the arms. The very high cervical regions, such as the AO or AA joint, can cause referred **retro-orbital** (behind the eye) pain or pain in the jaw. Your physician will try to help determine which joints are involved through your history and physical examination. However, not all pain syndromes follow a perfect pattern, and the specific joints involved must be confirmed with **diagnostic injection(s).**

Individuals suffering from a facet-related problem will typically have mechanical-type pain that is worsened by specific motions. In the cervical region, pain typically increases when looking to one side or the other and/or looking up or down. In the lower back, patients typically have pain when arching their back backwards. In the thoracic area, where there is much less movement, pain typically occurs with rotation (twisting) motions or sometimes with coughing and sneezing. During physical examination, feeling the joints (**palpation**) typically causes increased symptoms in the injured area. This finding is often used to identify which areas are to be injected.

Facet joints can be treated using two basic techniques. In the first technique, **intra-articular injection,** a needle is placed directly inside the joint (intra-articularly) to inject local anesthetic and steroid. A second technique, called a **medial branch block** or MBB, involves blocking or injecting local anesthetic with or without steroid onto the medial branches, which are tiny nerves that provide sensation to each facet joint. Two nerves (medial branches) **innervate** each facet joint, one from the level above and one from the level below. For example, to numb the C4–C5 facet joint, both the C4 and C5 medial branches are injected. Similarly, in the thoracic region, each joint can be injected intra-articularly by placing a needle inside the joint (which is often very difficult to accomplish in the thoracic region) or by blocking the medial branches of that level and the level above. The specific location of the medial branch in the thoracic region is highly variable, depending on whether it is the high-thoracic, mid-thoracic, or lower-thoracic region. Placement of the needles for these medial branch blocks requires an intimate knowledge of the location of the medial branch in a given location. In the lumbar region, some patients will have associated **sacroiliac joint injuries** (see chapter 12) and may require simultaneous or combined treatment of the lower lumbar facets and sacroiliac joints to achieve optimal relief. When both the facet joints and sacroiliac joints are involved, this is sometimes referred to as **posterior joint syndrome.**

These injections provide both important diagnostic information and therapeutic benefit. If the above therapeutic interventions result in symptomatic relief, even if it is only temporary, then the doctor can be sure that your facet joints are the cause of your pain. The duration of the injections' effect will dictate your doctor's next step. If prolonged relief is achieved with the injections, intermittent steroid injections to the facet joints can be performed on an as-needed basis up to three to four times per year if necessary. If the patient is only receiving short-term relief, **radiofrequency ablation** or **cryoneuroablation** treatment to kill those nerves is an alternative option (see chapter 13).

## After the Procedure

Recovery from simple local injections and steroid injections to the facet joints usually takes about one to two days. Patients often experience almost immediate pain relief from the local anesthetic, followed by slight discomfort from the injection, then rapid improvement in their symptoms. Fortunately, the potential risks and complications from these procedures are quite minimal, primarily infection and bleeding. There is the small potential for nerve injury. However, the risks of nerve injury can be dramatically limited by using appropriate techniques.

Your physician will want a careful report from you about any pain following the procedure, both during what is described as the **local anesthetic phase** (the first few hours when the injection site is numb) and over the next several days to weeks as the steroids take effect. Depending on the degree of benefit and duration of effect, your physician will make a decision about the next appropriate treatment step. Consider keeping a pain journal, a simple notebook in which you write down how you feel every day. Most of us can't remember by Friday what we wore to work on Monday, so it is easier to have something to refer back to when your doctor asks you two weeks after your injection how well it worked. Consider scoring your pain on a scale from zero to ten with zero being no pain and ten being the most severe pain you can imagine. Then you can review the numbers and see if you gradually got better or if you got better right after the procedure but rapidly returned to your baseline pain level. Also write down if you notice any improvement in your activity level. For example, before your facet injection you may have had difficulty bending down to put on your socks in the morning. If after the injection you can perform this activity with relative ease, it is important to tell your doctor that information.

## Questions to Ask Before Your Facet Block:

1. Will this injection be performed under **fluoroscopic guidance**? **"Blind" facet joint injections**, especially in the neck, can be potentially lethal. They are also extremely inaccurate. Some people are experimenting with **ultrasound** for facet joints, but the evidence of the safety and efficacy of that technique is not yet clear. Most insurance companies agree that "blind" injections are ineffective, and so they will not pay for them. For safety and accuracy, all spinal injections in IPM should be performed with radiologic guidance.

2. What approach or technique will you use?

3. At what level will the procedure be performed?

4. Will you use sedation? Do I need sedation?

5. Are there any restrictions after the procedure?

6. What complications can occur?

## Before the Procedure:

1. Make sure your doctor is aware of all medications you're taking. Some heart medications are **blood thinners** and will increase the risk of bleeding complications. In order to safely perform the facet block, these medications may need to be stopped for a certain amount of time before the procedure (at the discretion of the physician providing you with those medications). You may

also need to go for blood work the morning of the procedure to make sure your blood is clotting properly.

2. If you are diabetic, you must tell your physician ahead of time. **Insulin**-dependent diabetics will have to follow specific protocols before and after the injection. If you are having your procedure with sedation, you will need to fast before the procedure and you should bring your insulin with you to the procedure. You may also have some variations in your blood sugar levels for up to two weeks from the steroids in the injection. If you are diabetic, it is important that you monitor your blood sugar more closely for two weeks after the injection (or until your blood sugar is back under control). If you have a problem getting your blood sugar back into a normal range, consult the doctor managing your diabetes.

# CHAPTER 12

## SACROILIAC INJECTIONS: ANOTHER COMMON CAUSE OF BACK PAIN

The **sacroiliac joint** is the joint where the pelvis meets the tailbone (figure 4.7). This joint can be injured through **degeneration** or become painful following a lumbar fusion, when extra stress is placed on the joints below the surgical level (i.e., an L5–S1 fusion). The sacroiliac joint is also commonly injured in slip-and-fall accidents when the patient lands on his or her butt, or in a motor vehicle accident when the injured party presses one or both legs firmly against the floor just prior to impact (figure 4.8). After such traumatic injuries, the joint can become unstable and slip in and out of position. Finally, inflammation called **sacroiliitis** can occur in association with various rheumatologic conditions such as **ankylosing spondylitis**, **psoriatic arthritis**, and **Reiter's syndrome** (otherwise known as reactive arthritis).

Physical therapy is the cornerstone of treatment for sacroiliac joint dysfunction and will typically include manipulation and mobilization of the joint as well as stretching the surrounding muscles, such as the gluteal, piriformis, and quadratus lumborum muscles. Numerous muscles attach in and around the sacroiliac joint, as well as ligamentous structures that can be affected by injuries in this area (see figures 12.1 a and b).

If symptoms persist in the sacroiliac region despite conservative measures, consideration can be given to intra-articular sacroiliac joint injections. In this situation, a physician places a needle into the joint under direct x-ray guidance. Dye is injected to ensure the needle is placed within the joint (figure 12.2), followed by an injection of local anesthetic and steroid. If this results in symptomatic relief, it provides both therapeutic and diagnostic information. Your physician's next step will depend on the duration of benefit. If these injections provide relief for a reasonable amount of time, they can be repeated intermittently. If they don't provide prolonged benefit, alternative therapies may be considered.

**Radiofrequency ablation (RFA)**, cold RF ablation, or **cryoneuroablation** of the nerves that go to the sacroiliac joints (the **posterior** sacral rami or lateral branches) can provide symptomatic relief of sacroiliac joint pain (see chapter 13). If the sacroiliac joint is unstable, procedures that result in long-term stabilization of the joint can be considered. Conservative approaches include the use of prolotherapy in which a deliberately irritating medication or substance is injected to stimulate an inflammatory reaction, which the body responds to by growing new tissue in the area (see chapter 15). This serves to strengthen the **ligament** and tendinous structure and thereby stabilize the joint. In very rare situations, surgical sacroiliac joint fusions have been performed. This is a very aggressive approach with mixed outcomes and should be reserved for the most extreme cases.

# CHAPTER 13

## RADIOFREQUENCY ABLATION AND CRYONEU- ROABLATION: MAKING THE PAIN STAY AWAY

**R**adiofrequency ablation (RFA) uses electrical energy to kill nerves. Special insulated needles are placed on the nerves, and the physician then uses low-level electrical stimulation to identify the location of the target nerve. Once that nerve is identified, a small amount of local anesthetic is injected to numb the area, and then the nerve is heated with radiofrequency energy to interrupt its ability to conduct the pain signal. Radiofrequency ablation treatments typically last six months to a year, though some patients experience relief for several years. Note that RFA is reversible (it simply wears off when the nerve grows back) and can be repeated when the symptoms recur. Radiofrequency ablation can be used from the C2 level to the S1 level for **facet joints**, and there are several techniques now described for the **sacroiliac joint** as well.

**Cryoneuroablation**, or nerve freezing, is a similar technique that uses cold instead of heat. Under local anesthetic, a probe is placed on top of the nerve and localized with a peripheral nerve stimulator. The temperature of the probe's tip then drops to minus 70 °C, destroying the nerve but leaving the nerve insulation intact so the nerve can grow back along its normal path. This outpatient procedure can return the nerve to its normal function and give long-term relief. It is usually used on larger nerves; because the cold will kill the nerve but won't damage the insulation of large nerves, the nerves can grow back along their normal pathways instead of hitting scar tissue that can develop after surgery, RFA, or chemical nerve blocking with alcohol or **phenol**. The probe is much larger, so the area will be sore for several days after the procedure but because the nerve can grow back normally, a return to normal, pain-free function is possible. Cryoneuroablation, or "cryo," can be repeated if symptoms recur. Still, most doctors don't favor this technique, probably because they have never been trained in it. Also, no one has shown one approach to be superior to the other. RFA is generally felt to last longer and requires a much smaller needle, and cryo is not really a viable option in the cervical region because of the size of the probe that must be used.

Whichever technique is used, cryo or RFA, the physician will use low-level electrical stimulation to identify the location of the target nerve. This means you must be awake enough to give the physician feedback about how close the needle or probe is to the nerve (sort of like playing "Marco Polo" or "Hot, Warm, Cold"). Success with these treatments is dependent on the patient providing accurate feedback during the procedure.

After a nerve-destruction treatment, patients often experience some increased pain for approximately one week, followed by slow and progressive improvement over a six- to eight-week period. Some patients feel a burning sensation described as similar to sunburn, associated with light touch sensitivity after the procedure. This typically resolves over four to six weeks, and significant discomfort can be treated with creams, patches, and/or pills. Some patients have residual muscular spasm following these treatments. If this occurs, your physician may suggest treatment directed at the muscles (stretching and/or trigger point injections, see chapter 7).

# CHAPTER 14

## ADHESIOLYSIS: WASHING AWAY THE SCAR TISSUE

In chapter 10, we discussed epidural steroid injections, which can be a very effective technique to treat **chronic pain**. When epidural steroids are injected, the medicine moves along the path of least resistance; in certain circumstances this can prevent medicine from getting where it is needed. After surgery it is common for the **epidural space** to be clogged with scar tissue (adhesions), which can prevent medicine from reaching the inflamed nerve where it is needed. This scar tissue can usually be seen easily on MRI imaging that has been done with gadolinium (contrast) enhancement. Evidence of this is also found during epidural injections when contrast flow is blocked to the nerve by dense adhesions.

Scar tissue that has grown in the epidural space can wrap around a nerve and cause chronic irritation of the nerve which the patient will usually experience as chronic leg pain in the distribution of that nerve. You can develop adhesions in the spine as a result of surgery, infection, chronic irritation (such as with stenosis, a narrowed area in the spinal column), or in reaction to the chemical irritants from a chronically **leaking disc.** Sometimes these adhesions can be broken up quite easily, especially if it is soon after surgery, but other times the adhesions can be very dense and thick, making them more difficult to remove. Breaking up or removing these adhesions is called **adhesiolysis** (figures 14.1 a and b).

One of the techniques to deliver medicine to the desired area is to place a **catheter** inside the epidural space, steer it to the intended target area, and use fluid and medications to open up the blocked areas. An interventional pain physician, Gabor Racz, originally developed the technique and it is sometimes called a "Racz procedure." Because the catheter is sometimes difficult to steer, a steerable handheld device can be placed inside the tailbone and advanced to the target area. On the end of this hand piece is a flexible catheter that can be used to sweep back and forth and mechanically open up adhesions ("Navicath"). It is also possible to place a tiny fiber optic camera through a catheter, inside the spinal column (spinal endoscopy), which allows direct visualization of the nerves and provides arguably greater ability to break up adhesions under direct vision. To date, no study shows one of these techniques to be more effective than the other.

A variety of medicines can be injected in the epidural space. The most common is a time-released steroid, a depo-steroid. In the case of adhesiolysis, your physician can also inject a scar-softening medicine as well as a high concentration of salt solution to shrink the nerves and potentially kill the tiny pain nerves inside the spinal column.

Although this is a more invasive procedure than a simple epidural steroid injection and has slightly greater risks, it is less invasive than open back surgery and may be worth considering before undergoing a riskier open procedure. Open surgical resection of scar tissue has an extremely low long-term success rate (on the order of 5% to 10%) because patients typically develop recurrent adhesions, which are often worse than the original scar tissue. With the techniques described above, most studies suggest a success rate of 25% to 50%, although several have had even better results. With this approach, scar tissue is less likely to recur as compared to an open surgical technique; but if it does, this procedure can be repeated. You can always consider a more aggressive open surgery if **percutaneous** adhesiolysis doesn't work, but you may not be able to try this less invasive procedure if you decide to start with the more aggressive open surgery. Adhesiolysis should at least be considered before implantable techniques (e.g., spinal cord stimulation, see chapter 20) as it may prevent the need for this more involved, risky, and expensive surgery. Note that scar tissue that is more than a few years old is usually very difficult to break up. Your doctors may just move to the next step and elect to forgo adhesiolysis if that's the case due to the low success rate with that scenario. Be sure to discuss all your treatment options with your physicians so you can make an informed decision before undergoing this procedure.

## Risks and Complications

All procedures have risks; the more aggressive the technique, the greater the risks. Adhesiolysis is more aggressive than regular epidurals, and there are greater risks involved. When trying to peel apart the layers of adhesions, it is possible to tear one of the layers lining the **spinal canal** (the dura). Spinal fluid can leak out, causing a spinal headache. Local anesthetic could leak into the spinal fluid and cause very profound numbness, in other words a very high spinal anesthetic. Direct mechanical trauma to the nerve roots can occur, and if pressure inside the epidural space is too great, it could decrease the blood flow to the spinal cord itself or create increased spinal fluid pressure all the way up to the brain and the blood vessels going to the eyes. For this reason, it is critical that you are alert enough to tell your doctor if you are having any problems such as numbness, weakness, headaches, or changes in vision during the procedure. As with any procedure, there is a risk of bleeding or infection.

## Questions to Ask Before Your Adhesiolysis:

1. Will you use a catheter or a camera?
2. Will I need sedation?
3. Did my MRI and/or my previous dye studies with my earlier injections show a problem with dye spread from scar tissue?

# CHAPTER 15

## REGENERATIVE THERAPY: REBUILDING THE BODY'S NORMAL TISSUE

Most of what you have read so far has involved diagnosis and management of chronic painful conditions. However, just like changing tires on a car with bad alignment, this does not treat the underlying issue (the bent frame). The car will run better for a while, but the accelerated wear and tear on the tires will continue. Similarly, when musculoskeletal structures are unstable or out of alignment, they will cause secondary problems in surrounding structures. Pain is often caused by the instability that occurs with **ligament** or tendon laxity, strain, or tearing. Ligaments are fibrous connective tissues that attach one bone to another, and tendons are the tissues that attach muscles to bone. Loose ligaments can be associated with excessive motion and the development of pain. Muscles then must overwork and subsequently reside in a state of spasm to hold structures together and make up for the loss of normal tendon and ligament function; this leads to muscle pain and fatigue. Once an injury has occurred, if it is not adequately healed, the tissues holding structures together never return to their former strength. For example, a simple sprained ankle can be "weak" forever and prone to frequent re-injury.

Unlike a car, if we can slow down the degenerative process, our self-healing system might actually be able to reverse the wear and tear process. When you cut yourself and it gets red and swollen, this redness is from increased blood flow and the delivery of specific cells into the area for repair of the associated damage. The repair cells, called **fibroblasts**, lay down new tissue to reinforce the torn or damaged tissue. Inflammation triggers this response, just like

75

a piece of sand stimulates an oyster to lay down mother of pearl. Regenerative therapy involves the injection of growth factors onto tendon and ligament attachments and stimulates a local inflammatory reaction in the area of injection. This stimulates the body to repair itself. Tightening down ligaments and improving the attachment of muscles on the bones restores the stability and strength of the musculoskeletal system, which hopefully will improve both function and pain, the goal of all pain therapies. Although not covered by most insurance today, these techniques may actually be the cure that you have been looking for.

Regenerative therapy (originally called fibroproliferative therapy and now called prolotherapy) attempts to stimulate the production and activation of fibroblasts at the attachment of ligaments and tendons. The goal is to induce a natural healing process to strengthen these structures. The technique was developed in the 1930s as a nonsurgical treatment for hernias and became popular in the 1950s. It became very popular among general practitioners, but unfortunately, because of their lack of training, several patients were seriously injured, which gave the technique a bad reputation. The technique began to flourish again in the 1990s.

Newer approaches have emerged over the last five to ten years that involve the injection of a patient's own blood products onto the tendon attachment. Chemicals released from platelets, tiny cell fragments in the blood that help with clotting, trigger fibroblast proliferation. The most effective injections have the highest concentration of platelets and therefore the highest concentration/ amount of tissue growth factors. In this newer approach, blood is removed from the patient and then placed in a centrifuge to separate the plasma and various cells. The platelet rich plasma (PRP) is then injected onto ligament and tendon attachments. PRP is being injected into knees, hips, and elbows of professional athletes and even injected into the face by plastic surgeons to "tighten up" the tissues like a facelift.

**Stem cells** are the ultimate healing cells. You have heard a great deal about stem cells from embryos, but you also have stem cells in your bone marrow, the blood-cell factories inside your bones. These cells can be sucked out of your bone marrow, cultured, and then re-injected into the injured structures. Recently, stem cells were also identified in the fat cells that lie underneath your skin, called **adipose tissue.** One of the newest regenerative techniques involves sucking out fat cells from the belly, mixing them with a chemical that stimulates the growth of stem cells, and then injecting that solution onto the injured tissues. Imagine a liposuction that would get rid of your knee pain!

Regenerative therapy requires a comprehensive look at the injury, with a careful and thorough examination of the surrounding structures, to best understand how the interactions of one body part may be affecting other adjacent or connected structures. Factors that must be considered for treatment of any musculoskeletal injury include alignment, stability, and neuromuscular function. Understanding the proper musculoskeletal function of the body and how various structures interact is essential to planning regenerative therapy treatments.

# CHAPTER 16

## DISCOGRAPHY: A BETTER LOOK AT YOUR DISCS

If your doctor is recommending a **discogram**, you are probably pretty far along in treatment and have already tried a variety of simpler injections for your pain. In fact, discography should rarely, if ever, be offered as the primary or first intervention. Discography is an invasive test with a greater degree of risk than many of the other simple diagnostic and therapeutic procedures discussed earlier. With that said, for a patient who needs a discogram, it can be a valuable diagnostic tool.

Discography is a highly specific diagnostic test that has no therapeutic value but can provide useful information about the anatomy of the disc and help the physician to determine which disc is the cause of your pain. Needles are placed into multiple **discs** within a specific region of your spine (cervical, thoracic, or lumbar). The discs are then injected with dye (contrast) to increase the pressure inside the disc, which distends the center of the disc and places pressure on its outer wall where the nerve endings are located. Discs that significantly reproduce the "usual pain" at low pressures are felt to most closely correlate with those that are causing pain on a daily basis. (Discography is more likely to reproduce back pain than leg pain.)

Other useful information is obtained about the disc's anatomy both from the fluoroscopic images during the actual discogram and from the **CT scan** that typically follows. Discography always requires the injection of more than one disc because at least one level must serve as a control level, that is, a disc that should not be painful during provocative testing. Once the needles are properly positioned, the physician then injects the discs in a random order while asking the patient what he or she feels at each level (figure 16.1). The order is random to keep you from unconsciously allowing the information you have about your injury to affect your responses. For example, if every doctor you have ever seen has told you that you have a herniated disc at L4–L5, if the physician performing the discogram told you that he was injecting L4–L5 you may tense up because you expect that disc to hurt, or you may believe that level will hurt more and express discomfort even if the disc is not actually painful. This doesn't mean that you're crazy or that the doctor thinks you're going to lie or exaggerate. When we expect something to hurt, we tense up and anticipate the worst. The random testing order removes the bias created by how you think the discogram is going to feel.

Injecting dye into the disc distends the disc and increases the pressure, which allows the physician to test how each disc feels when it's loaded, or pressurized. A level that reproduces the patient's pain, or at least a component of the patient's pain, is considered a positive discogram, or concordant.

Pain can be caused by two main issues: a tear in the disc allows the fluid within the disc to leak out, which irritates the nerve endings of the disc's outer wall; or the disc has a herniation (like a bubble on the sidewall of a tire) and the distension of the disc from pressurization causes increased compression of the surrounding tissue. When dye is injected into the disc, the resulting pressure should reproduce your pain in a location and pattern similar to your usual symptoms; the goal of discography is to determine which discs reproduce which part of your pain. More than one disc may be positive on discography, which would indicate that more than one may be causing the different components of your pain. The degree or level of pain that is reproduced is usually moderate to severe.

By definition, discography is therefore a painful test, and as we initially noted, it has no beneficial therapeutic effects. In fact, patients often will experience an increase in their pain for about a week following discography. However, the diagnostic information can be crucial to the workup and treatment of back or neck pain. Because the most important part of this test is determining what the patient feels during the pressurization of the disc, the patient must be alert and responsive to accurately report what he or she is feeling as the disc is pressurized. Even if sedation is utilized it will be light so the patient can provide accurate reporting. Placing the needles is usually accomplished without significant discomfort, especially if the patient can relax during needle insertion.

## Risks and Complications

Discography is not without risk. The physician will be placing needles in the vicinity of nerves, so there is a risk of nerve injury, although it's small and usually avoidable with care and attention. One of the more concerning risks is that of infection. Because discs do not have good blood flow, infection in a disc can be very difficult to treat. Your physician will likely give you **prophylactic antibiotics** through one or two different approaches to reduce the risk of infection.

Recently it has been suggested that discography may accelerate disc **degeneration**, but this has not been substantiated in large-scale studies. Most physicians who perform discography do not believe this to be the case based on many years of experience and following many patients who have previously undergone discography.

Discography is an important diagnostic procedure that can help to clarify the extent of damage and provide a different view of the inside of your disc to show a clear picture of the cause of pain. This information assists physicians in making decisions about your treatment.

# CHAPTER 17

## MINIMALLY INVASIVE DISC SURGERY: WHEN LESS IS MORE

Minimally invasive sounds good, right? It sounds like an easier surgery, and in many ways, it is. This type of procedure is an alternative to open back surgery. Some clinicians look at these less invasive and less damaging approaches as the future of spine surgery. It is not appropriate for everyone, and the key to a successful outcome lies in your physician making sure you are an appropriate candidate.

Minimally invasive disc surgery represents a combination of various therapies designed to treat injured and/or damaged **discs** within the spine. These are most commonly performed for lumbar (lower back) injuries; however, some physicians also perform these treatments in the cervical (neck) and thoracic (mid-back) areas. In general, these procedures treat one of two different types of disc pathologies or injuries. The most common injury treated with this procedure is a **disc herniation** or **disc bulge**. In this situation, the disc protrudes or sticks out beyond the confines of the normal disc, like a bubble in the sidewall of a tire (figures 5.2 a and b). If it is in the right (or wrong) place, the disc herniation can compress and irritate a nerve within the spine (figure 4.2). Once the herniation is removed, the cause of the irritation goes away, and the pain goes with it. So how do we get rid of the herniation?

There are many types of **percutaneous disc decompression** surgeries; some work by removing material inside the disc (intradiscal approach), but this technique can only be used with a **contained herniation**. Other percutaneous techniques work on the outside of the disc (extradiscal approach) and may be appropriate for more complex disc extrusions. Intradiscal decompression decreases the pressure inside the disc and provides room for the herniation to move back into the disc space. This procedure is performed percutaneously (through the skin) and involves the removal of disc material through a needle, or **cannula**. A variety of techniques and approaches are available. The majority of these therapies remove disc material from the **nucleus**, or center, of the disc. Today there are many new procedures (and more being developed) to remove disc material percutaneously from within the **spinal canal** and **neural foramen** (the hole where the nerve exits).

All **intradiscal techniques** (surgery that occurs inside the disc) remove material from the center of the disc (the **nucleus pulposus**). When your doctor chooses this approach, he or she may mechanically cut out material with a variety of devices or simply vaporize the tissue, which turns it into gas that can leak out through the needle. Your doctor will review your films to determine where your herniation is located on the disc and in the canal, its shape, and the size of your disc (its height from top to bottom). Then he or she will assess any surrounding **degeneration** and damage before deciding if percutaneous removal is appropriate and which technique is most likely to help you. This requires that your physician have experience in reading MRIs, **discograms**, and **CT scans**. The technique your doctor chooses will depend on what your herniation looks like and what he or she is most comfortable with as an operator.

Intradiscal percutaneous discectomy approaches include **Nucleoplasty®** (figure 17.1 c), Disc Dekompressor® (figure 17.1 f), **LASE** (laser assisted spinal endoscopy, figure 17.1 e), **Nucleotome®** (figure 17.1 a), **percutaneous endoscopic discectomies**, and several other approaches. The different therapies each work via a different mechanism to remove disc material. These procedures only work for "contained" herniations. This means the herniation must be attached to the disc, not a free fragment, and that it must be contained by the back wall of the disc (the **annulus**, see chapter 4) and not ruptured through that outer wall. The herniation also must be of a specific size and shape for these approaches to be successful. Discs that have collapsed beyond 50% of their normal height, or those with a significantly **extruded herniation**, typically can't be treated via percutaneous intradiscal approaches. (However percutaneous extradiscal approaches may be appropriate for large disc extrusions).

**Disc tears** are also commonly treated percutaneously. In this situation, the disc has a crack or tear in its outer wall. The body reacts to this injury by growing small blood vessels into the area. Unfortunately, with these blood vessels grow small nerve endings. The center of the disc contains chemical irritants that can leak out through a tear and irritate the small nerve endings. This causes what is referred to as **discogenic pain**: the disc itself hurts. Good candidates for repairing discs with tears will have otherwise relatively healthy discs (i.e., the discs must still have at least half their original height from top to bottom). Patients with discs that have significant associated end-plate damage, bony instability (**spondylolisthesis**, where one bone slips out of position in relation to the bone above or below), and/or the presence of a significant compressive disc herniation would not be good candidates for this procedure. Some physicians combine percutaneous decompression of the disc with repair of the annulus to treat both components of the damage.

Repair of the disc's outer wall can be accomplished with a therapy called IDET® (**intradiscal electrothermal annuloplasty**). In this procedure, a coil is threaded around the inside of the the the annulus (figure 17.1 d). Once positioned, the coil is heated using radiofrequency energy, which serves two theoretical purposes; to repair the tear in the outer wall of the disc and to denervate the disc so that it can no longer be painful (similar to an RF for **facet joints**). It is likely that repair of that outer wall of the disc occurs through the creation of organized scar tissue, similar to regenerative therapy, in reaction to the heat injury. A newer approach called **Biacuplasty®** (figure 17.1 g) is emerging, and it is unclear at this time whether it will be more or less effective than IDET®. Several other approaches are on the horizon for repairing annular damage, but these have not been fully studied at the time of this first edition. We hope in later editions to provide you with more information on these emerging technologies.

The major advantage of these therapies for the patient is that, since they are less invasive, they cause less tissue damage to other adjacent structures such as bone and muscle, which should equate to a quicker recovery and reduced risk. Perhaps their biggest advantage is that they can help the patient avoid more aggressive and risky surgery. Open surgical disc decompression and treatment typically involves removal of some of the **ligament** and bony structures of the spine. Unfortunately, this can lead to later destabilization of that spinal segment. Instability can cause increased and abnormal motion of that spinal segment and usually is associated with pain.

If the back pain is severe enough, some patients undergo spinal fusion surgery to prevent that movement. Fusion surgeries are unfortunately associated with less predictable outcomes and have a significant chance of making things worse (some estimate this at 10-20%). Avoiding the risk of spinal destabilization reduces the risk of a more aggressive surgery. When it comes to back problems, less is often more. Most pain physicians view open spinal surgery as a necessary evil: sometimes it's needed, but it should be avoided whenever possible. We know several spine surgeons who have refused fusion surgery for themselves because of its risks, preferring to find other ways to manage their problem.

Other minimally invasive techniques have recently been developed for the removal of overgrown ligaments in the back of the spine. As we age, the joints and ligaments of the spine grow in response to the stresses of normal life activities. When these grow too much, it can cause a condition called **spinal stenosis** (as was discussed in chapter 4) with associated nerve compression. For patients who do not respond on a sustained basis to epidural injections and where the stenosis is primarily related to **ligament flavum** overgrowth, percutaneous removal is now an alternative to open surgery. The procedure, called minimally invasive lumbar decompression (MILD), is still new, but early studies look promising.

The minimally invasive techniques discussed in this chapter are indicated for both young and old patients, as long as the individual patient's spinal anatomy is appropriate for the planned approach. If there's a chance that a percutaneous procedure will help you, it's probably worth giving it a try, since percutaneous procedures don't burn bridges. You can always have open back surgery if the percutaneous procedure doesn't work, but you can't go back and try the percutaneous procedure if the open procedure doesn't work. Putting off that first open surgery as long as possible prevents or at least delays the need for a fusion. Since a fusion at one level can put pressure on adjacent disc levels, this can also delay the progression of disc disease at other levels. By preventing the first operation, you may prevent or at least delay the need for multiple operations later, especially for someone with multilevel disc disease. Unfortunately, many insurance carriers, including Medicare, do not approve of these newer and less invasive therapies.

## Side Effects and Complications

The most common complications with this type of surgery include **discitis** (infection of the disc), nerve injury, and/or bleeding. The incidence of these complications is very low (less than 2%). To limit your risk, you should expect certain things from your physician. Any work performed on a disc should be performed in a completely sterile environment. Intravenous antibiotics, sterile prepping, and sterile technique are mandatory for the safe performance of these treatments. Because these surgeries are uncomfortable, sedation is usually provided.

If symptoms persist after minimally invasive disc surgery, your physician may recommend further epidural and/or facet injections if there is residual inflammation around the nerve roots in the **epidural space** or a secondary problem with the facet joints. This doesn't necessarily mean that the minimally invasive disc surgery was unsuccessful; it indicates that other pathology is present that requires additional treatment. Most minimally invasive disc surgery is performed intradiscally (inside the disc), so it doesn't change pre-existing nerve inflammation inside the spinal canal, a condition that may require epidural steroid injection or adhesiolysis therapy (see chapters 10 and 14). Some patients will have residual back pain that requires treatment related to the arthritic component (facet-related symptoms) of their spinal degeneration.

## After the Procedure

Following minimally invasive disc surgery, patients should expect a period of recovery. Be realistic; although this is a less invasive procedure, someone is still operating on your disc. Your body needs time to recover. You're not going to wake up the next morning and be able to move boulders. You should expect a period of increased symptoms for approximately one week for each level that is treated; for example, a patient with two-level surgery should expect some increased pain and soreness for about a two-week period. The symptoms in the legs or arms will typically improve over about a one-month period, and pain in the lower back will typically improve over a two- to four-month period. Between four to eight weeks after surgery, your physician will likely recommend a course of physical therapy including a spinal stabilization program, which works by strengthening the core musculature. It's essential that you cooperate with this program and commit to an exercise regimen that will improve your spinal stability for the long-term health of your spine. Odds are if you made it to this point, your back has been hurting for a while. This means you have limited your activity level. The muscles you once used all the time have become deconditioned and need to be strengthened. **Spinal decompression** therapy may also aid in healing and remodeling of the disc as it heals.

## Questions to Ask Your Doctor:

1. How many levels will you address with minimally invasive surgery?
2. How long will I be out of work? (This will depend on what type of work you do.)
3. Which techniques will you use?
4. How many of these procedures have you performed?
5. What is your success rate?
6. What complications have you seen?
7. What are my other options? If you want to know about the conventional surgical options, then ask to be referred for a consultation with a qualified surgeon.

## Before the Surgery:

1. Provide your physician with copies of your latest MRI or CT scans.
2. You physician may request that you wear a back brace for a period of time after your surgery. It is best to obtain this in advance and bring it with you to the procedure.

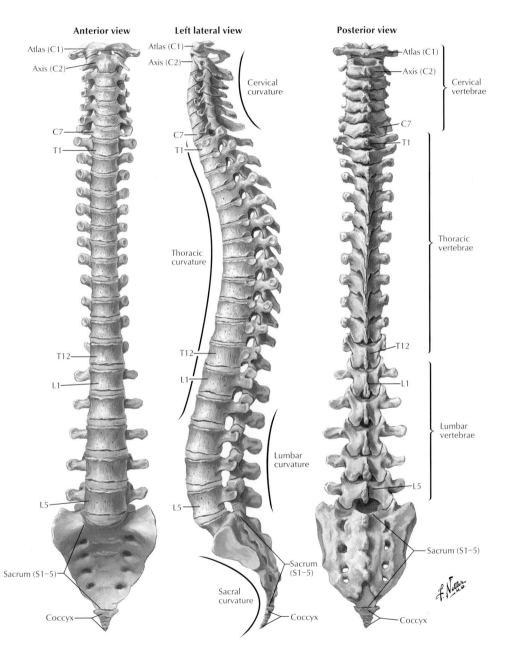

**Anterior view**

Atlas (C1)
Axis (C2)
C7
T1
T12
L1
L5
Sacrum (S1–5)
Coccyx

**Left lateral view**

Atlas (C1)
Axis (C2)
Cervical curvature
C7
T1
Thoracic curvature
T12
L1
Lumbar curvature
L5
Sacrum (S1–5)
Sacral curvature
Coccyx

**Posterior view**

Atlas (C1)
Axis (C2)
Cervical vertebrae
C7
T1
Thoracic vertebrae
T12
L1
Lumbar vertebrae
L5
Sacrum (S1–5)
Coccyx

## Figure 4.1

Spinal anatomy from neck to tailbone.

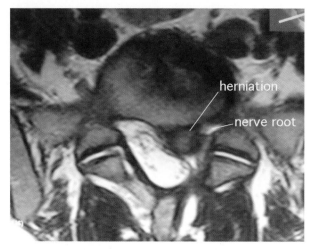

**Figure 4.2**
Disc herniation pushing on a nerve.

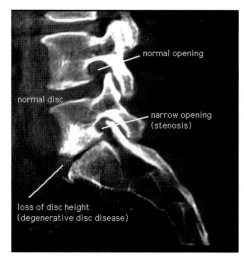

**Figure 4.3 a**
Foraminal or nerve opening stenosis.

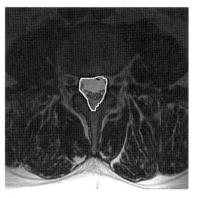

**Figure 4.3 b**
Normal central canal size (a white line is drawn around the margins of the spinal canal).

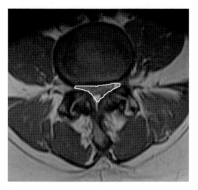

**Figure 4.3 c**
MRI showing central and lateral recess stenosis (a white line is drawn around the margins of the spinal canal).

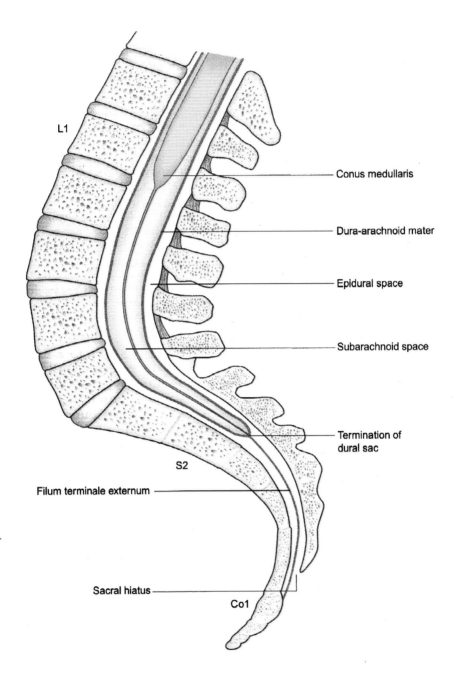

L1

Conus medullaris

Dura-arachnoid mater

Epidural space

Subarachnoid space

Termination of dural sac

S2

Filum terminale externum

Sacral hiatus

Co1

**Figure 4.4**
Epidural space and contents.
Reproduced from *Gray's Anatomy, 39th ed.*, Susan Standring, Copyright Elsevier (2005).

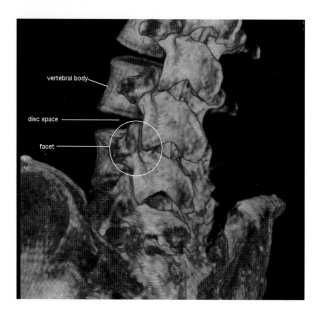

vertebral body

disc space

facet

**Figure 4.5**
Facet joints.

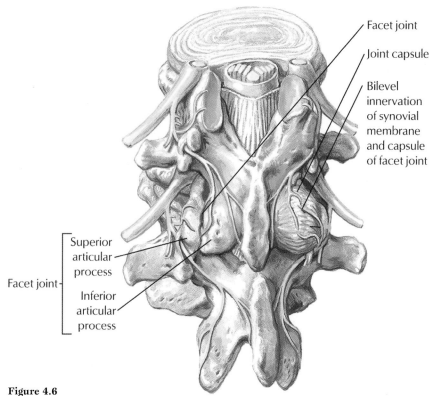

Facet joint

Joint capsule

Bilevel
innervation
of synovial
membrane
and capsule
of facet joint

Superior
articular
process

Facet joint

Inferior
articular
process

**Figure 4.6**
Facet nerves.
Courtesy of The American Society of Interventional Pain Physicians, from Manchikanti et al.
*Interventional Techniques in Non-Spinal Pain, 2009,* ASIPP Publishing, Paducah, KY

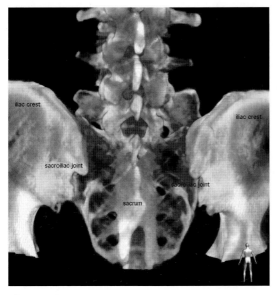

**Figure 4.7**
Sacroiliac joint.

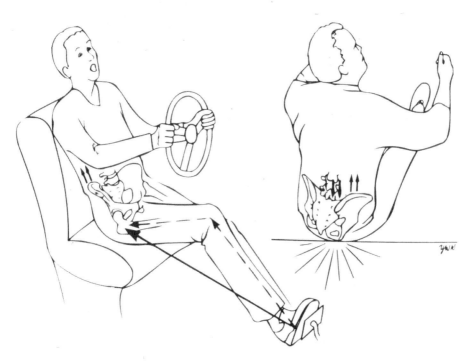

**Figure 4.8**
Mechanisms of sacroiliac joint injury from car accident or slip and fall.
Used with permission from *Ligament and Tendon Relaxation Treated by Prolotherapy.* Beulah
Land Press, 2002, Oak Park, IL.

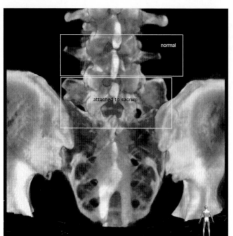

**Figure 4.9**
An abnormal overgrowth of bone on side of the spine attaching part of the lowest vertebral body to the sacrum. (This is a common congenital abnormality known as a transitional segment.)

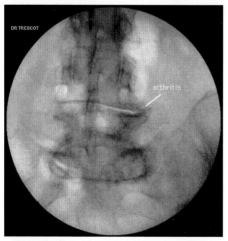

**Figure 5.1**
Low back x-ray showing an abnormal overgrowth of arthritic bone on one side of the spine ("bone spur").

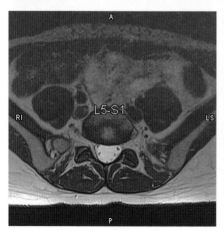

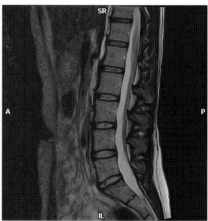

**Figures 5.2 a**
MRI lumbar spine showing mild disc bulging, cross section or axial view.

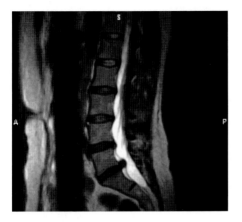

**Figure 5.2 b**
MRI (herniated disc)—head-to-toe slice (sagittal).
Disc herniation can be seen at the lowest disc level
(black structure protruding into white spinal fluid).

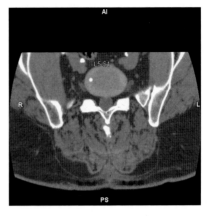
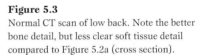

**Figure 5.3**
Normal CT scan of low back. Note the better
bone detail, but less clear soft tissue detail
compared to Figure 5.2a (cross section).

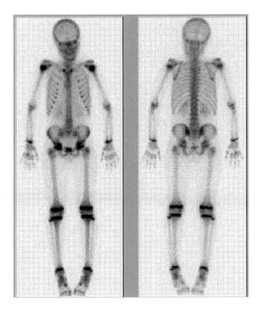

**Figure 5.4**
Bone scan. Dark areas represent areas of arthritis.

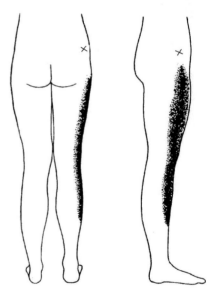

**Figure 8.1**
Trigger point pattern of pain that mimics in
distribution the lower extremity radiating
symptoms that are seen with a disc herniation but
for which there is a different cause.(X = trigger
point, shaded area is the distribution where the pain
is usually experienced.)

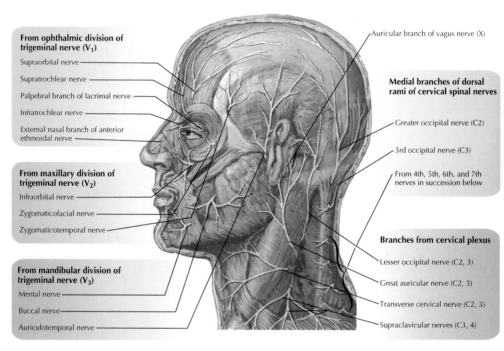

**From ophthalmic division of trigeminal nerve ($V_1$)**

Supraorbital nerve

Supratrochlear nerve

Palpebral branch of lacrimal nerve

Infratrochlear nerve

External nasal branch of anterior ethmoidal nerve

**From maxillary division of trigeminal nerve ($V_2$)**

Infraorbital nerve

Zygomaticofacial nerve

Zygomaticotemporal nerve

**From mandibular division of trigeminal nerve ($V_3$)**

Mental nerve

Buccal nerve

Auriculotemporal nerve

Auricular branch of vagus nerve (X)

**Medial branches of dorsal rami of cervical spinal nerves**

Greater occipital nerve (C2)

3rd occipital nerve (C3)

From 4th, 5th, 6th, and 7th nerves in succession below

**Branches from cervical plexus**

Lesser occipital nerve (C2, 3)

Great auricular nerve (C2, 3)

Transverse cervical nerve (C2, 3)

Supraclavicular nerves (C3, 4)

**Figure 9.1**

Nerves of the head and face.

2011. Used with permission of Elsevier. All rights reserved.

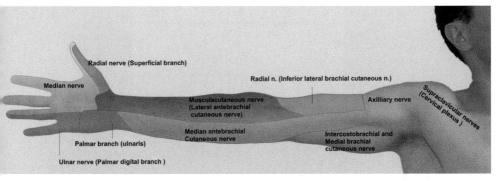

**Figure 9.2**

Nerves of the upper extremity.

(Hadzic, A., Vloka, J., *Peripheral Nerve Blocks,* ©2004, McGraw-Hill) Reproduced with permission of The McGraw-Hill Companies.

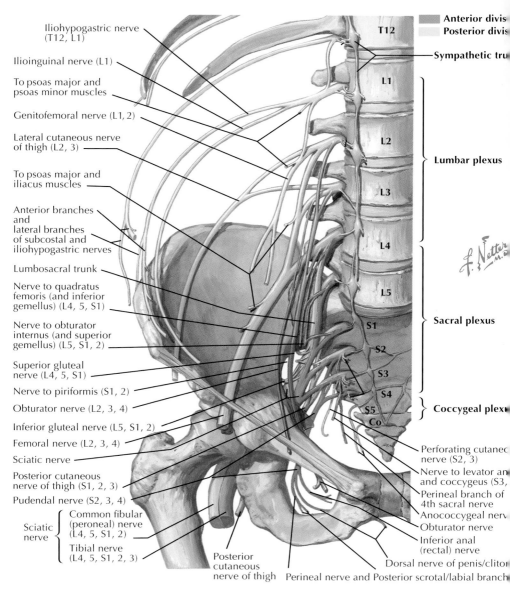

Iliohypogastric nerve (T12, L1)

Ilioinguinal nerve (L1)

To psoas major and psoas minor muscles

Genitofemoral nerve (L1, 2)

Lateral cutaneous nerve of thigh (L2, 3)

To psoas major and iliacus muscles

Anterior branches and lateral branches of subcostal and iliohypogastric nerves

Lumbosacral trunk

Nerve to quadratus femoris (and inferior gemellus) (L4, 5, S1)

Nerve to obturator internus (and superior gemellus) (L5, S1, 2)

Superior gluteal nerve (L4, 5, S1)

Nerve to piriformis (S1, 2)

Obturator nerve (L2, 3, 4)

Inferior gluteal nerve (L5, S1, 2)

Femoral nerve (L2, 3, 4)

Sciatic nerve

Posterior cutaneous nerve of thigh (S1, 2, 3)

Pudendal nerve (S2, 3, 4)

Sciatic nerve {
Common fibular (peroneal) nerve (L4, 5, S1, 2)
Tibial nerve (L4, 5, S1, 2, 3)
}

Posterior cutaneous nerve of thigh

T12

L1

L2

L3

L4

L5

S1

S2

S3

S4

S5

Co

Anterior divis
Posterior divis

Sympathetic tru

Lumbar plexus

Sacral plexus

Coccygeal plex

Perforating cutaneo
nerve (S2, 3)

Nerve to levator an
and coccygeus (S3,

Perineal branch of
4th sacral nerve

Anococcygeal nerv

Obturator nerve

Inferior anal
(rectal) nerve

Dorsal nerve of penis/clitor

Perineal nerve and Posterior scrotal/labial branch

### Figure 9.3

Nerves of the chest, abdomen, and pelvis.

ILIOLUMBAR LIGAMENT
SUP CLUNEAL NERVES
SUP GLUTEAL NERVE
PIRIFORMIS
GREATER TROCHANTER
SCIATIC NERVE
ISCHIAL TUBEROSITY

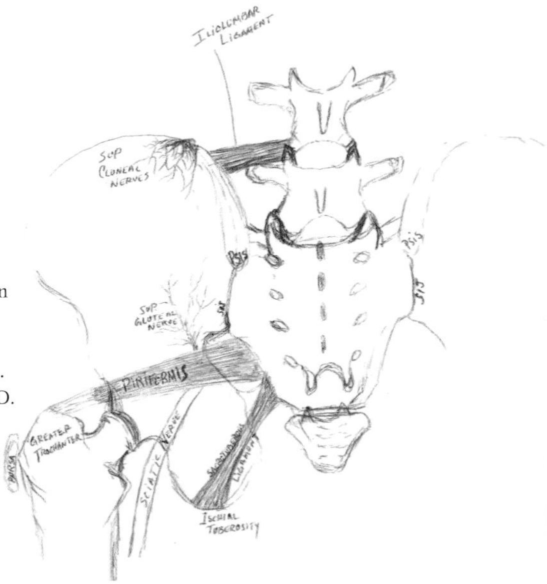

**Figure 9.4**
Many different structures can cause pain to refer into or down the leg; this is referred to as "pseudosciatica". This diagram shows some of these structures.
Credit: Luis N. Hernandez, M.D.

cluneal
sacral
superior gluteal
sciatic

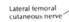

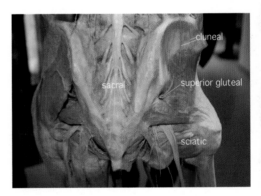

**Figure 9.5**
Nerves of the back and sacrum.

Lateral femoral cutaneous nerve
Anterior cutaneous branches of femoral nerve
Infrapatellar branch of saphenous nerve
Medial crural cutaneous branches of saphenous nerve
Cutaneous innervation

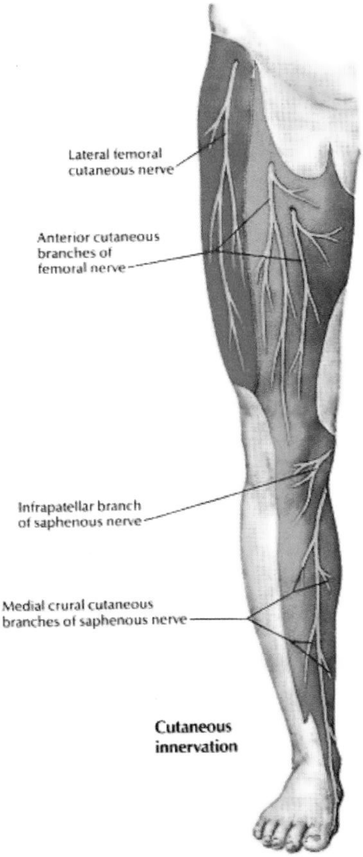

**Figure 9.6**
Nerves of the lower extremity.
Courtesy of The American Society of Interventional Pain Physicians, from Manchikanti et al. *Interventional Techniques in Non-Spinal Pain,* 2009, ASIPP Publishing, Paducah, KY

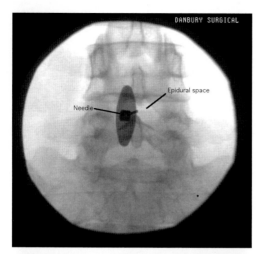

**Figure 10.1 a**
Lumbar interlaminar epidural (front to back view).

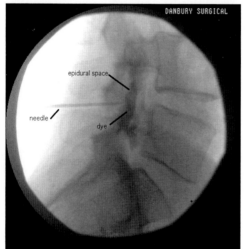

**Figure 10.1 b**
Lumbar interlaminar epidural (side view). Needle positioned in epidural space, dye has been injected and is spreading in the posterior epidural space.

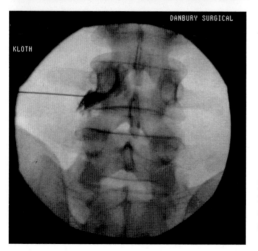

**Figure 10.2**
Lumbar transforaminal epidural. Dye spreading along nerve root and proximally into the lateral recess of the epidural space.

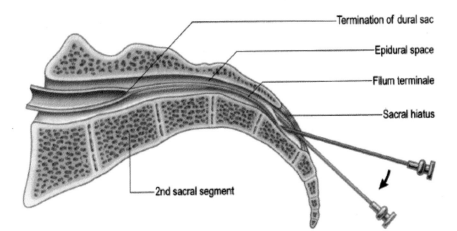

**Figure 10.3 a**
Caudal epidural injection.
Reproduced from *Gray's Anatomy, 39th ed.*, Susan Standring, Copyright Elsevier (2005).

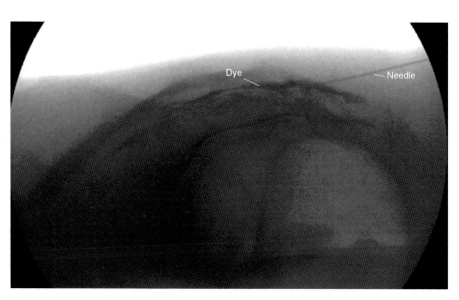

**Figure 10.3 b**
Caudal epidural injection x-ray. Needle positioned in the caudal canal with dye spreading in the epidural space (lateral view).

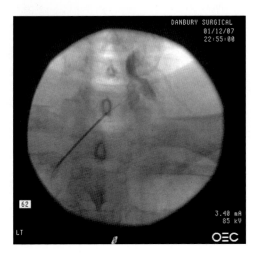

**Figure 10.4**
Cervical epidural with catheter technique, see dye spreading along the nerve after it exits the tip of the catheter.

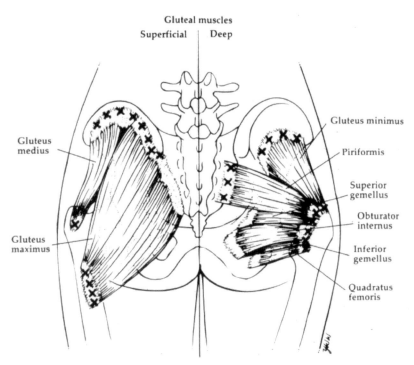

**Gluteal muscles**

Superficial | Deep

Gluteus medius

Gluteus maximus

Gluteus minimus

Piriformis

Superior gemellus

Obturator internus

Inferior gemellus

Quadratus femoris

**Figure 12.1 a**
Muscles around the sacroiliac joint.
Used with permission from *Ligament and Tendon Relaxation Treated by Prolotherapy*. Beulah Land Press, 2002, Oak Park, IL.

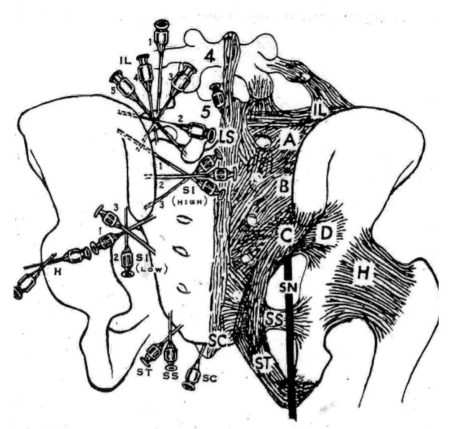

**Figure 12.1 b**
Ligaments around the sacroiliac joint.
IL = iliolumbar ligament
SS = sacrospinatus
ST = sacrotuberous
SI – sacroiliac
SN = sciatic nerve
Used with permission from *Ligament and Tendon Relaxation Treated by Prolotherapy.* Beulah
Land Press, 2002, Oak Park, IL.

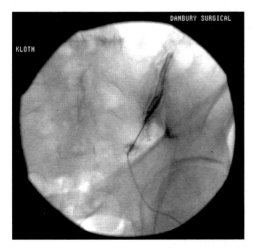

**Figure 12.2**
Sacroiliac joint injection (dye seen spreading
along the inside of the joint space).

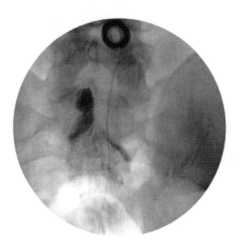

**Figure 14.1 a**
Adhesiolysis. (Note filling defect on the right at the tip of the catheter.)
Manchikanti L, Singh V (ed). *Interventional Techniques in Chronic Spinal Pain.* Pg 495. 2007, ASIPP Publishing, Paducah, KY.

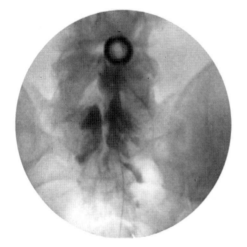

**Figure 14.1 b**
Adhesiolysis. Note dye filling the defect after the scar tissue has been broken up (lysed).
Manchikanti L, Singh V (ed). *Interventional Techniques in Chronic Spinal Pain.* Pg 495. 2007, ASIPP Publishing, Paducah, KY.

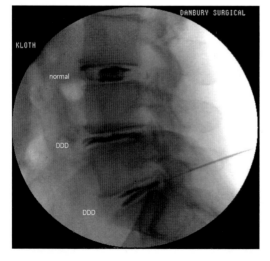

**Figure 16.1**
Discogram. Note dye spreading within the disc, the three discs show varying degrees of degeneration as evidenced by the variable pattern of dye spread within the disc.

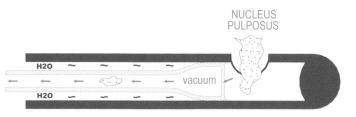

NUCLEUS PULPOSUS

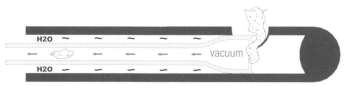

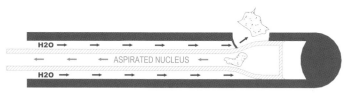

**Figure 17.1 a**
Nucleotome. A reverberating blade within the cannula cuts off pieces of disc that are vacuumed into the cannulas side wall.
Photo provided courtesy of Clarus Medical.

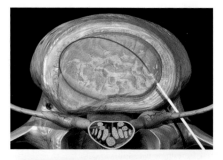

**Figure 17.1 b**
Acutherm. The ACUTHERM™ Decompression Catheter features a heating coil designed to treat disc bulges or herniations directly. ACUTHERM™ Targeted Disc Decompression compliments of NeuroTherm.

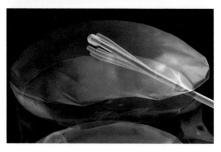

**Figure 17.1 c**
Nucleoplasty. This procedure removes disc material by creating channels within the disc using radiofrequency energy, vaporizing disc material which leaves the needle as a gas. Photo provided courtesy of ArthroCare® Corporation.

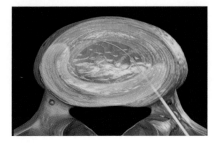

**Figure 17.1 d**
IDET. By inserting the SPINECATH™
Intradiscal Catheter into the annulus of the
affected disc, physicians can apply controlled
levels of thermal energy to treat cracks and
fissures in the disc.
SPINECATH Intradiscal
ELECTROTHERMAL™ Therapy compliments
of NeuroTherm.

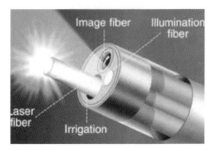

**Figure 17.1 e**
LASE. LASE allows direct visualization of the
inside of the disc to assist with mechanical
decompression using both a laser and grasping
forceps to remove disc material from the
nucleus.
Photo provided courtesy of Clarus Medical.

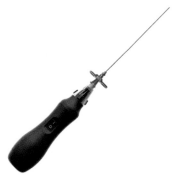

**Figure 17.1 f**
Dekompressor. This procedure uses a rotating
wand with screw-type threads positioned along
the tip. The threads catch the disc material and
then pull it back into the needle for removal of
disc material.
Photo provided courtesy of Stryker
Interventional Spine.

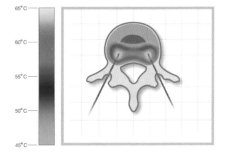

**Figure 17.1 g**
Biacuplasty . This procedure involves placing one
needle into each side of the disc and then creating
an area of radiofrequency energy between the
needles to seal annular tears and denervate the
inner annulus between the needles.
©Kimberly-Clark Worldwide, Inc. Used with
permission.

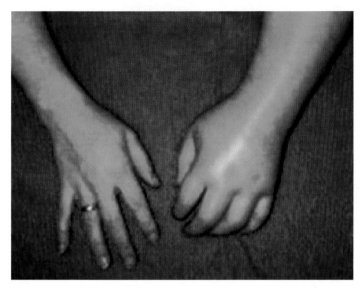

**Figure 18.1**
Chronic regional pain syndrome (CRPS) of the left hand. (Note shiny skin, swelling and discoloration.)

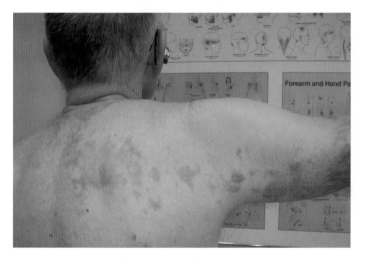

**Figure 19.1**
Acute herpes zoster or shingles. (Note rash in a band-like distribution extending from the back into the upper arm, following a right T2 distribution.)

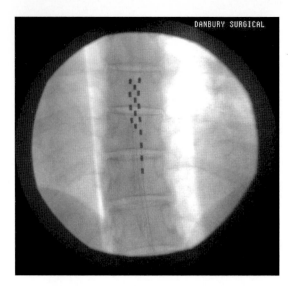

**Figure 20.1**
Spinal cord stimulator (three leads positioned in the spinal canal to treat back and leg pain).

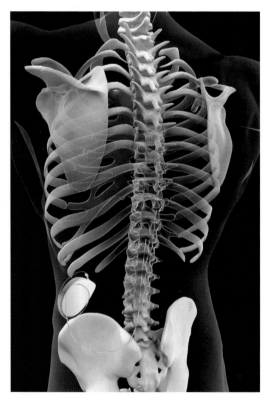

**Figure 20.2**
Spinal drug delivery system. Note pump in the left abdomen with a catheter (yellow line) running from the pump, around the flank, and then into the spinal canal.

*Courtesy of Medtronic, Inc.*

# CHAPTER 18

## COMPLEX REGIONAL PAIN SYNDROME: ONE SMALL NERVE CAUSING BIG PROBLEMS

**C**omplex regional pain syndrome (CRPS) is a **chronic pain** problem that most people don't even know about unless they or a friend or family member has it. CRPS is one of the most difficult and painful chronic pain conditions to treat and is associated with severe burning pain and hypersensitivity to touch. This condition usually follows a nerve injury; your doctor will try to identify the specific injury because it may hold the key to successful treatment. The causes of CRPS are beyond the scope of this book and are actively debated within the medical community.

Patients with CRPS frequently describe burning, stabbing pain that is associated with sensitivity to touch. It can be difficult to understand the needs of a person suffering from CRPS. They often seem anxious and are frequently scared that someone or something will touch the affected area. Consider your hand for a moment. Right now you are holding a book and touching the page. But think about all the things that touch your hand that you have minimal control over. When you take a shower, the water hits your skin; when you sleep, your hand touches the sheets; and in the winter, you wear gloves. Imagine being unable to tolerate any of those things because the least amount of pressure causes extreme pain.

In addition to pain, patients frequently describe color changes in the extremity, describing it turning blue and cold or red and hot, along with swelling and sensitivity (figure 18.1). These are called **vasomotor changes** and are evidence of the misfiring of nerves (sympathetic nerve dysfunction). **Sympathetic nerves** are a component of the autonomic nervous system, which automatically and without your conscious participation controls many different functions within the body. This includes sweating, hair erection, pupil size, heart rate, bowel function, and many other important bodily functions that are done without conscious control. These nerves are supposed to turn on if you're injured, but in people with CRPS, they never turn off again. If you stick your hand in a fire, the nerves in your hand produce a burning sensation so you know to pull your hand out of the fire before you seriously damage it. Once you pull your hand out of the fire, that sensation should go away. Someone with CRPS experiences that moment of pain but the pain signal never turns off, or it becomes so sensitive that the least amount of stimulation feels like the hand is back in the fire.

## Treatment for Complex Regional Pain Syndrome

The cornerstone of CRPS treatment includes exercise, physical therapy, and increased use of the involved area, even though that's very painful. Treatment of the injured peripheral nerve that caused the CRPS, when it can be identified, can be highly effective. **Antiseizure** medicines seem to help because these medications stabilize nerves and prevent excessive firing, similar to how they treat seizures. Seizure medications stabilize the nerve membranes and decrease their firing rate; calming the nerve firing decreases pain and the nerves become less sensitive. **Antidepressants** and a variety of other medications can also be very helpful to control the pain.

When symptoms persist beyond these conservative measures, early intervention with injections that temporarily shut down the sympathetic nerves can be effective for this pain syndrome, sort of like rebooting a computer. The literature clearly supports that the earlier these interventions are performed, the more likely they are to be successful. The physician must diagnose this condition as early as possible.

Unfortunately, in some patients all of these measures fail, and those patients may ultimately need to undergo more aggressive treatment in the form of implantable therapies (see chapter 20). Spinal cord stimulation is most commonly used, which replaces the pain signal with a soothing tingling sensation. This therapy is best described as a distraction therapy: nerves can only carry one signal at a time, so the tingling sensation produced by spinal cord stimulation prevents the pain signal from getting through to the brain. As a last resort, consideration could be given to an implanted drug delivery system. Both of these modalities should be preceded by a trial of that type of interventional therapy, described in more detail in chapter 20.

## Sympathetic Blocks

There are three types of nerves: feeling (sensory) nerves, muscle (motor) nerves, and sympathetic nerves. Unlike the motor and sensory nerves that travel along very specific routes, the sympathetic nerves travel as a net all over the body, and they gather together in several places called **ganglia**: the neck, the belly, the lower back, and at the tip of the tailbone. Placing local anesthetic on one of those gathering spots, or ganglion, is called a sympathetic ganglion block and is most commonly used for the treatment of CRPS conditions. Intermittent injections are typically used, but a pain physician can alternatively create a continuous sympathetic blockade using an epidural **catheter** or by placing a catheter along the indicated sympathetic nerves. The pain physician can attempt to aggressively treat CRPS by using either intermittent daily injections or a continuous infusion for a period between one week and three months (depending on the clinical situation and the response to therapy). Note that not all cases of CRPS are sympathetically mediated and therefore some forms of CRPS ("non-sympathetically mediated") cannot be controlled with sympathetic blocks.

In the cervical region, sympathetic blocks are typically performed at the **stellate ganglion**, which is a collection of nerves in the sympathetic chain that sit in the front of the neck at approximately C7 to T1. The cervical sympathetic chain can actually be injected in a number of locations along the sympathetic chain, but physicians typically do this at C6 or C7. Some physicians will block these nerves at T2 or T3. The thoracic levels require an approach from the back.

Stellate ganglion blocks were performed for years without **fluoroscopic guidance** by feeling for a specific bony bump in the front of the cervical region. Today, these injections are typically performed with fluoroscopic guidance for accuracy and safety. The thoracic approaches require a much greater degree of caution due to the potential risk of a **pneumothorax** (collapsed lung). Although this risk also exists for the cervical or neck approaches, it is a much lower risk than it is with a thoracic approach. Certain precautions must also take place for any patient undergoing a stellate ganglion block because local anesthetic can spill on to the phrenic nerve that **innervates** the **diaphragm**, an important muscle for breathing. Because of this, stellate ganglion blocks should never be performed on both sides at the same time. The physician must take this risk into account before performing this injection for a patient with pulmonary compromise (i.e., severe lung disease) or other associated breathing problems, and it may be too dangerous for some patients.

In the lumbar region, the sympathetic chain lies along the anterolateral border (front side) of the spine and extends predominantly from L2 to L4. These nerves are approached by placing needles from the back side of the spine toward the front surface of the spine.

**Celiac plexus** and other abdominal sympathetic blocks are typically used for cancer pain management but have been used by some physicians for the treatment of chronic **pancreatitis** and other abdominal conditions. This collection of sympathetic nerves lies in front of the **aorta** (the biggest blood vessel in the abdominal region). Approach of this ganglion requires specific training for this procedure and a full awareness of the potential risks and complications. With that said, this is a relatively safe procedure that has a very high success rate for the treatment of abdominal pain from certain conditions such as pancreatic cancer. In fact, it is the first-line treatment for patients with abdominal pain from pancreatic cancer who don't respond to oral medications.

Pelvic pain conditions including **interstitial cystitis**, chronic pelvic pain, **radiation neuritis**, and other pelvic injuries can sometimes be treated with superior and inferior **hypogastric plexus** blocks. This set of sympathetic nerves lies in front of the L5–S1 juncture and again requires specific training and expertise in order to place a needle safely in this region. A collection of sympathetic nerves at the very tip of the spine in front of the tailbone region (called the **ganglion impar**) can be blocked for the treatment of certain types of rectal pain, most typically stemming from cancer or its associated treatments.

In addition to blocking sympathetic nerves directly at the sympathetic ganglion, these nerves can also be more centrally blocked in the **spinal canal** by performing an epidural. In fact, multiday sympathetic blocks can be achieved by placement of catheters in the **epidural space** and then re-injecting these on a daily basis; this can also be performed by placing catheters along the sympathetic chains, although epidural catheters seem to be more stable in their position in most patients. In some patients with particularly severe pain, a continuous epidural infusion can be used for one week up to three or four months for treatment of severe complex regional pain syndrome. During that period of continuous sympathetic blockade, the patient should also undergo aggressive physical therapy treatment to improve function and range of motion. Sympathetic discharge causes blood vessels to constrict, think of it as a way of the body self-preserving and protecting an injured area. If that area is bleeding out, constriction of the vessels will limit the extent of blood loss. Sympathetic discharge causes redirection of blood to vital organs to protect the body. So with a sympathetic discharge the patient's affected area will often turn pale, due to constriction of the blood vessels to that area. When you block the sympathetic nerves, the area receives increased blood flow and turns red. This can lead to a decrease in blood pressure as the body redirects the blood volume to a larger area. When blood is distributed to more areas, there is less in the major blood vessels (we all have a fixed amount of blood in our systems) and can lead to a drop in blood pressure.

# CHAPTER 19

## POST-HERPETIC NEURALGIA (PHN): EARLY TREATMENT IS THE KEY TO SUCCESS

Chickenpox (herpes varicella) is an extremely common childhood disease. Many of us remember the painful itchy sores that guaranteed us a week out of school while we soaked in oatmeal baths and tried not to scratch. Not as many people are familiar with the disease's adult counterpart, shingles (herpes zoster), until they have experienced this painful disease. It is estimated that one in ten individuals who have had chickenpox will develop shingles and this disease strikes 200,000 to 800,000 patients in the United States each year. Shingles is most commonly seen in the elderly population and people who are immunosuppressed.

Shingles can begin in the way that you normally feel when you contract the flu, except this virus is followed by a painful rash. Initially people often report feeling run down or as if they are coming down with something a few days before the blistering rash appears. Many people experience pain, itching, tingling, fever, fatigue, and/or muscle pain prior to developing the rash. Unlike the chicken pox where the rash appears all over the body, the shingles rash generally appears on only one side and in one dermatome (i.e. in the distribution of a specific nerve; on the chest this appears as a horizontal strip). The rash usually begins as an area of redness and then blisters develop (figure 19.1). Towards the end of the second week the blisters begin to crust over and dry up. The crust usually falls off by the third to fifth week leaving behind pink scars that can become numb and light colored. The most common areas for shingles to appear on the body are the thoracic area (around your mid-section, belt line, bra line, etc.) or in the trigeminal nerve area (face and head). Shingles can also appear in the lumbar area (low back) and sacral area (tailbone), but this is rarer.

After experiencing an episode of chicken pox, the virus that caused the infection settles down to live in your nerve cells for the rest of your life. These virus particles lie dormant inside the cell body, near the spine, until one day when the virus decides to reactivate. This seems to occur at times when the immune system is not working its best, such as during stress (why Mom told you to take care of yourself, stress and fatigue can make you more prone to infection), older age, or in those with disease-induced immunocompromise, such as someone with cancer or HIV.

Inside the body, the shingles virus spreads when active virus particles travel down the course of an involved nerve root. The blisters, or vesicles, form at the very end of the nerve, where they terminate at the level of the skin; these blisters contain active (live) viral particles. It's the presence of the viral particles in the blisters that makes this disease contagious at this point in time. Patients with oozing blisters must be very careful to avoid contact with pregnant women and anyone who has not had the chicken pox. The chicken pox virus can be extremely dangerous to adults and the unborn child.

Post herpetic neuralgia (PHN) refers to the nerve damage that can linger long after the shingles virus has cleared. When the virus travels down the nerve it causes inflammation and hence **edema** formation (swelling) of the nerve. This swelling can compromise the blood supply to the nerve, which can lead to the death of parts of the nerve. If you were to look at a cross section of a nerve affected by PHN under a microscope you would see that there was a loss of the larger nerves. These larger diameter fibers are the part of the nerve responsible for normal sensory function, the small diameter neurons that remain are the nerves responsible for transmitting pain sensation. Large diameter neurons have an inhibitory influence on the small diameter pain-transmitting neurons. The loss of this sensory input from the large diameter neurons at the level of the **central nervous system** causes PHN.

The good news for most shingles patients is that only 20-30 % of people who get shingles develop post herpetic neuralgia. The risk for developing post herpetic neuralgia increases with age. While it is almost unheard of for a 20-year-old patient with shingles to develop post herpetic neuralgia, somewhere around 50-75 % of patients over the age of 70 who have shingles will go on to develop PHN. This dramatic increase occurs because older patients are more likely to have pre-existing vascular disease, which would exacerbate the effect of the compromised blood supply to the affected nerve (similarly, I have found younger patients with vascular disease to be at higher risk as well). Symptoms can range from a mild burning sensation to a more severe pain that is so bad patients can't stand to have anything (including clothing) touching the affected area. Light touch sensitivity is one of the hallmarks of this condition.

For patients that develop acute shingles, the most important part of their treatment may be early intervention to prevent progression to a full-blown PHN. Patients who receive the appropriate treatment within the first four weeks of their shingles outbreak have a greater than 90% chance of avoiding a permanent post herpetic neuralgia. The success rate for treatment decreases with time; the farther out from the date of initial outbreak that the patient receives treatment, the poorer the results. Patients who receive treatment during the second month have an 80% success rate. Patients who wait more than two months to seek treatment have only a 20% success rate and patients who wait a year for treatment have only a 5% success rate. Clearly, early intervention is the key to a successful outcome.

There is a very distinct difference between treating shingles and preventing or treating post herpetic neuralgia. Patients with shingles will often be prescribed antiviral medication, which will help fight the active infection and reduce the infectious period. These medications will often accelerate the healing time for the rash and help dry up the blisters. There is no evidence however that antiviral agents will reduce the risk of PHN, a condition that is best prevented, rather than treated later. Therefore, in addition to treating the active infection, we must consider who is most at risk for developing PHN and then try to treat those individuals early, to prevent the possible associated nerve damage and long-term chronic burning pain that accompanies PHN.

While post herpetic neuralgia can be treated with medications such as **anticonvulsants**, tricyclic **antidepressants**, and oral narcotics, these are usually only partially effective and often the severe light touch sensitivity and burning pain persists. If the pain doctor sees you early enough, it is likely that they will recommend a nerve block to help reduce the pain and, as importantly, to help the nerve heal without permanent nerve damage. Nerve blocks have been hypothesized to help improve nerve blood supply and thereby help prevent nerve death. What procedure to perform is dependent on the location of the shingles on your body and how long it has been since your outbreak. In milder cases the doctor might do a onetime injection, whereas in more severe cases they may recommend a series of injections over a one- or two-week period.

The more pain there is during the acute shingles outbreak, the more it seems patients are likely to develop significant PHN and so the more aggressive your doctor will likely be. If your shingles outbreak is on your face or head, the injection may be in your cervical spine, if you have shingles in the chest area, the injection may be in your thoracic spine (mid-back), etc. For patients with more aggressive PHN, the doctor may choose to insert a **catheter** to allow for multiple repeat injections or even a continuous infusion of local anesthetic. The catheter may stay in for about a week and after the last injection is performed, the doctor will remove the catheter.

Some patients do not achieve long-term relief with nerve blocks and in these individuals further attempts at medication management should be considered. Intra-lesional injections have been advocated by some, as has Capsaicin treatment. If severe pain persists, a trial of spinal cord stimulation may be considered. This intervention for PHN has, at best, a 50 % success rate and is reserved for the more extreme cases.

# CHAPTER 20

## IMPLANTABLE TECHNIQUES: SPINAL CORD STIMULATION SPINAL DRUG DELIVERY SYSTEM PERIPHERAL NERVE/FIELD STIMULATION

You and your doctor by now should have a pretty good understanding of what is causing your severe **chronic pain**. Maybe you have tried several of the other treatments described elsewhere in this book but still have disabling pain that limits your functional capacity. Or perhaps the other treatments you have tried, like high-dose medications, were associated with significant side effects that limited your function. Implantable techniques involve insertion of a semi-permanent device into the body to control pain and may be an option to consider at this point. Implantable therapies work by acting on the nervous system to block or distract from the sensation of pain and are referred to broadly as neuromodulation therapies.

## Spinal Cord Stimulation

One alternative your doctor might explore when other methods have failed is spinal cord stimulation (SCS) (figure 20.1). This therapy involves the application of microcurrents of electricity to certain areas of the spinal cord. The most common use of SCS in North America is to treat pain. However, in Europe these devices are used to treat blood flow insufficiency, usually in the legs, but sometimes even in the heart. No one knows for certain how SCS really works, although there are several well-developed theories. In selected cases it can be remarkably effective at relieving pain and improving functional capacity.

SCS produces a sensation of tingling in the painful area of the body that changes the way pain is perceived. Sometimes referred to as a distraction therapy, SCS seems to block or alter the perception of pain at the level of the **central nervous system** (brain and spinal cord). You may be familiar with **TENS (transcutaneous electrical nerve stimulation)** units or interferential units with pads that you wear over the painful area of the body, but SCS is something entirely different. If you've tried TENS (a less invasive, topical form of electrical stimulation) and haven't had success with that therapy, don't assume SCS won't work for you. In fact, there is no meaningful correlation between whether TENS helps or not and the effectiveness of SCS (or, for that matter, peripheral nerve stimulation).

SCS was developed for the treatment of neuropathic (nerve) pain. This pain is typically associated with injury to nerves and is described by patients as burning, shooting, or tingling. It may be associated with other neurologic changes like painful numbness or a greatly increased sensitivity to things that would not normally produce pain, such as light touch. For example, diabetes can attack nerves in the arms and legs and produce a severe burning or tingling sensation that might be associated with numbness and pain. This kind of pain typically does not respond well to narcotic pain relievers. When it was first used in patients, SCS was more or less restricted to the treatment of purely neuropathic pain of the arms or legs. Recent advances in technology have made it more useful for the management of pain in other areas of the body, such as in the back or pelvis.

**Getting Started with Spinal Cord Stimulation**

This therapy is not for everyone. First of all, it involves having a medical device implanted into your body. Although some physicians advocate earlier use of this modality, most will at least attempt a more conservative treatment approach and only turn to SCS if those methods fail to achieve adequate relief for the patient.

Like spinal drug delivery systems, SCS systems are expensive, so the Medicare program and most major insurers require a psychological evaluation to screen for conditions that can limit this therapy's effectiveness. You will have to perform a trial before the permanent implant is inserted. SCS trials typically last three to seven days. For the trial, your doctor will place wires through a needle into the **epidural space** and steer these to lie over specific areas of your spinal cord. During the procedure, you must be aware enough to answer questions about whether you feel stimulation and where you feel it. The doctor will try to find a position for the wires that allows electrical stimulation, perceived as a soothing tingling sensation, overlying the painful areas. Once a good location is identified, your doctor will secure wires, called leads, to your skin. A temporary external pulse generator (battery) will be attached to the end of the lead that's outside your body, and this is programmed to provide stimulation (a soothing tingling sensation) to the areas of the body where pain is experienced. A good way to think of stimulation techniques is as a distraction therapy; it covers up or masks the pain by giving the central nervous system a different sensation in the same area as the pain. There are eight different contacts on each lead, and each of those can be positive, negative, or off. You and your doctor literally have thousands of combinations available to optimize the stimulation pattern. You will carry this around with you during the trial period, and you will be asked to keep track of whether the stimulation relieves pain and what effect it may have on your ability to do your activities of daily living. At some point you and your doctor will then decide whether it makes sense to have one of these devices permanently implanted into your body. Depending on the particulars of your case and your doctor's local practice, the test procedure might be conducted by one doctor (an interventional pain physician) and the permanent implantation might be done by a spine surgeon.

## How it Works

The SCS system consists of a programmable (and usually rechargeable) pulse generator (the battery) that generates the individual and particular stimulation pattern for that patient. The generator is connected under the skin to leads that are placed in the **spinal canal** as described above. Your "mileage" on the battery will be determined by how often you use it and how high the settings are. Replacing the battery means replacing the entire pacemaker-sized pulse generator. The leads come in two types: those that can be placed through a needle (**percutaneous** leads) and those that are placed surgically (paddle leads). Paddle leads are more stable in terms of position and more energy efficient, but traditionally have been associated with the need for greater surgical trauma during insertion and hence a longer recovery period (recent developments may change this need for open surgery to place all paddle leads).

Both approaches have their merits and you should discuss these with your physician.

One advantage of SCS is that it gives you quite a bit of control. You will get a controller that works a lot like the remote for your TV. You can turn it on or off, select different therapeutic programs, and control the stimulation. Another major advantage of SCS is that it uses electricity instead of drugs, so there are no nasty side effects to speak of. In fact, many patients who use these systems find they can reduce their daily medication intake, and some can even eliminate medications altogether.

### Side Effects and Complications

As with any surgery, there are risks associated with implanting these devices. One of the most problematic is infection. Because these devices are a foreign body and therefore do not receive direct blood flow, an infection in your unit probably will not respond to treatment with antibiotics, and the system will likely have to be removed. You can have another device put in after the infection is completely resolved, but you might have to work with an infectious disease specialist the next time around.

Once you have an SCS system implanted, you generally can't have MRI examinations. The wires of the stimulator leads or the generator can heat up and theoretically cause damage. In some cases, you might be able to have an MRI of the head or an extremity in a special scanner, but otherwise a **CT scan** may be a reasonable substitute. Another potential problem with SCS systems is that the lead wires can migrate, which causes a loss in coverage over the painful areas and makes the device less effective than before. In some cases, the units can be reprogrammed to get the stimulation back. If reprogramming doesn't work, then the leads might require surgical repositioning. Other mechanical complications include lead fracture, which requires lead replacement.

## Spinal Drug Delivery Systems

A **spinal drug delivery system** infuses medicines directly into the spinal fluid and to the spinal cord. Cells that have a big influence on the perception of pain are located in the spinal cord, and this direct delivery can have a very potent and profound pain-relieving effect (figure 20.2). These benefits are achieved at total dosages that are much lower than it would take to get the same effect from pills, which limits side effects.

When you take pain medication by mouth, only a small portion of the drug molecules actually reach the sites in the brain and the spinal cord where they exert their powerful effects. Your liver metabolizes a lot of the medication before it can even get to where it's going, and your circulatory system sends those drug molecules everywhere in your body—even your hair—so it gets heavily diluted. Drug molecules that treat pain typically work on the central nervous system and have to penetrate the blood-brain barrier before they can exert their effect. These obstacles can sometimes be overcome by increasing the dose, but this also increases the side effects, including decreased cognition.

What if we could bypass the liver, the circulatory system, and the blood-brain barrier with a "smart bomb" of pain medicine? Well, about 30 years ago an **anesthesiologist** was getting desperate about one of his patients who had serious cancer-related pain, so he decided to try injecting morphine directly into the spinal fluid to see if it would help. And it did! It wasn't long before this discovery found its way into chronic pain management.

## Getting Started with Spinal Drug Delivery Systems

Before you get too excited you should know that these systems are not for everyone. Patients with persistent severe and disabling pain or who experience serious side effects from medications are the typical candidates for this type of therapy. Generally, a surgically implanted pump is a treatment of last resort and should only be considered in circumstances where just about everything else that can reasonably be done to treat the problem has already been tried.

It's very important to have realistic expectations about what this therapy can do for you. Most doctors consider this therapy successful if the patient can achieve at least 50% to 60% pain relief over a sustained period of time. As with any approach, it's usually just not realistic to expect 100% relief. After all, drug therapy doesn't solve the problem that produced the pain in the first place. It serves instead to change the perception of the pain that results from the condition.

This therapy is particularly expensive to start, but it's usually cheaper to maintain than oral medications. You could buy a nice car with the amount of money it takes to get the device implanted in the first place. And just like a car, it needs to be refueled periodically. Refills for the pump are generally cheaper in the long-run than pills, so these devices can ultimately result in an overall savings in health care costs. Because of the cost, Medicare programs and most insurance companies require a psychological evaluation and trial first (like a car, you get to take this out for a test drive before buying). In most cases a psychological examination will be required to screen for conditions, like severe uncontrolled depression, a factor that can be a barrier to effective pain management.

Your doctor will place medication into your spinal canal as a test to determine whether this therapy helps your pain. The trial period can last anywhere from a few hours up to about a week, depending on the technique your physician uses. Some patients find it helpful to write down their experiences during the trial period so they can compare it to their usual pain. If the trial period proves successful, you and your doctor may decide to place a more permanent system.

## How it Works

The system itself consists of a drug pump and a **catheter** that delivers medication directly into the spinal canal. Depending on the circumstances, the catheter can be placed in one of two locations in the spinal canal: the epidural space or the **subarachnoid** space. If the catheter is in the epidural space, the drug has to find its way across the dura to get into the spinal fluid. If the catheter is in the subarachnoid space, then the medication goes directly into the spinal fluid; this is known as an **intrathecal drug delivery system**. The vast majority of pumps deliver medications intrathecally because of the significant decreased dosage requirement (tenfold difference).

Permanent intrathecal drug delivery systems are totally implanted under the skin, both the pump and the catheter. You don't see the device directly, but the pump, which is about the size of a hockey puck, will be visible if you are thin and visit the beach. Your body size will determine how much it protrudes and how well you can hide the pump. A programmable pump can be reset by sending messages to the pump with radio waves, thereby allowing the physician to change the daily dosage without touching the patient.

Sometimes with cancer patients the catheter is placed into the epidural space and then attached to an external pump that you carry around with you (usually in a "fanny pack"). The useful life of an epidural system is shorter because they eventually become clogged or infected and have to be removed.

As of 2010, the Food and Drug Administration has officially approved three medications for use in these systems, but other medications are frequently and safely used to optimize pain control. Commonly used narcotic-type medications include morphine, dilaudid, fentanyl, and occasionally sufentanil. Other adjuvant medications frequently used include **bupivacaine** (a local anesthetic) that seems to help lower narcotic requirements, clonidine for neuropathic pain, and **baclofen** for muscular spasticity. Prialt® was the last intrathecal drug to be approved by the FDA, and is useful for neuropathic pain. It is extremely expensive and requires frequent refills; it should only be used when other medications are not effective.

## Side Effects and Complications

As effective as these spinal drug delivery systems can be, they can have side effects and complications too. There are risks associated with the anesthesia and surgery needed to get the device into your body in the first place. If the system becomes infected it's usually impossible to treat with antibiotics because the body cannot effectively fight the bacteria that accumulate on the surface of the implant; antibiotics can't be delivered by your body's bloodstream to the site of the infection, the implant or foreign body itself. If infection occurs, the system will probably have to be removed.

The side effects of the drugs used in these systems are pretty much the same as when these same drugs are administered by other means. However, because it's possible to get better pain relief with drugs given into the spinal canal at much lower dosages, you may find you have less severe side effects with a spinal drug delivery system. A commonly quoted rule of thumb is that you can get as much pain relief from one milligram of morphine delivered directly into the spinal fluid as you can from taking 200 to 300 milligrams a day by mouth!

There are two complications that are more or less specific to these systems. One is that delivering drugs in this way can produce persistent swelling in your ankles, called **edema**. Trying different drugs or combinations of drugs may be required to manage the problem. Some patients may need to take water pills to help them eliminate the extra fluid. In more severe cases, dosages may need to be lowered or the therapy discontinued. A second and common problem is hypogonadism or suppression of testosterone levels in the body (intrathecal narcotics can also effect estrogen levels but this is less common). Hypogonadism can occur in anyone receiving long-term, moderate to high dosages of narcotics via any delivery approach (oral, transdermal, or intrathecal). A less common problem is chronic urinary retention (difficulty emptying the bladder); this can also lead to fluid retention.

A more serious problem that can occur with spinal drug delivery systems is called a **catheter tip granuloma**. It doesn't happen very often but when it does, it requires urgent diagnosis and treatment. Under certain conditions, a mass of inflammatory cells and other material can form near the tip of the catheter as it sits in your spinal canal. If the mass gets big enough, it can result in compression of nerve roots and a progressive loss of pain relief. The physician needs to have a high index of suspicion and watch carefully for changes in neurologic function, loss of pain control, or the development of new pain symptoms. The most dependable way to diagnose this problem is to get an MRI and look for the inflammatory mass at the tip of the catheter. This means it has to be read by a radiologist who knows what your doctor is looking for. If you get a catheter tip granuloma and the problem is severe enough, you may need to have surgery to release the compression. More typically this is managed by turning off the infusion of medications through the pump, changing the fluid inside the pump to saline, and allowing the body to absorb the granuloma. Changing the catheter is always an option, but care must be taken during removal to prevent further spinal damage (the catheter can adhere to nerves or the spinal cord).

Doctors and pharmaceutical companies are always conducting research to develop better drugs that have fewer side effects. And the medical device companies are always looking for ways to produce better systems that have fewer complications. One concern that patients have about using this therapy is that they might not feel pain if they injure themselves. Don't worry. If you're doing something that is truly harmful, your body will let you know.

## Peripheral Nerve/Field Stimulation

Peripheral nerve stimulation (PNS) uses similar principles to SCS to treat pain. By stimulating **peripheral nerves** one can also provide treatment of a variety of painful conditions that affect a discrete localized area. Examples include **occipital nerve** stimulation for headaches, sacral nerve stimulation for pelvic pain, and subcutaneous field stimulation of the abdominal wall for treatment of post-herniorrhaphy pain.

With this technique, stimulating leads are placed near, or directly on, peripheral nerves to provide 'coverage' of the painful area. When subcutaneous nerve stimulation is utilized, some refer to this as field stimulation to separate it from direct peripheral nerve stimulation. In general, these are new areas of study, and much work remains in the study of this form of stimulation.

## Finding Additional Information

Medical device companies have educational videos that you can view to get more information about these treatments. You can also access their websites. Although you can't believe everything you read on the Internet, the best place to start your own investigation is to get approved information from a reputable company. Spinal cord stimulators are currently manufactured by three companies (Boston Scientific, Medtronic, and St. Jude Medical) and all three offer information on their devices. The most commonly used spinal drug delivery system is manufactured by Medtronic (a programmable pump), but several other companies make non-programmable pumps and several others are about to be released into the market.

# CHAPTER 21

## CANCER PAIN: EFFECTIVE CONTROL IS USUALLY POSSIBLE

When the subject of cancer is brought up, most people think of **chemotherapy**, radiation, the lost hair and weight, as well as the severe pain that can accompany this diagnosis. When someone has cancer, the first specialty that comes to mind is **oncology,** and that needs to be the guiding treatment whenever possible, but pain management also needs to be considered. With proper pain management, using the vast array of treatments available today, cancer pain can usually be controlled; however, accessing those treatment options isn't always easy. Because the well-intentioned oncologist concentrates on the disease and its potential cure, pain management often isn't fully addressed. Being informed and knowing what questions to ask improves your chance that these options will be made available.

Cancer pain is one of the more challenging areas of pain management. Many factors must be considered when deciding on a course of treatment. Some people need pain management to treat the side effects that arise from the cancer treatments. For example, neuropathic pain can result from radiation or chemotherapy-induced neuropathy (nerve damage). In some cases, the patient is left with a constant and painful reminder of the chemotherapy or radiation after the cancer is cured. Treating both the pain and the cancer requires great flexibility on both the pain physician's and oncologist's part to optimize coordination of care. For example, the timing of invasive treatments needs to be coordinated with chemotherapy schedules because chemo lowers the white blood cell count (which increases risk of infection) and lowers the platelet count (which increases the risk of bleeding). For the patient with terminal cancer, there are many other issues to consider when discussing pain treatment options, including how it will affect other long-term care needs. There are also multiple psychosocial issues surrounding the end of life that must be dealt with in a coordinated approach when planning and considering treatment alternatives. Some pain physicians prefer not to work with cancer patients because they have not had the training or experience to feel comfortable doing so.

With cancer, as with any other painful condition, it is extremely important to determine the precise cause of symptoms. Is the pain coming from a nerve being compressed or invaded by a tumor? Is it coming from tumor growth into soft tissue or adjacent structures? Is it distention of an organ? Or is it the growth of tumor into a bone and/or fracture of a weakened bone from tumor invasion? Determining the precise cause of the symptoms is essential to effective treatment.

Treatments for cancer pain can vary from the very simple to the very complicated. Some of these treatments carry incredible risk, and some are not even invasive. Less invasive treatments can include the use of radiation therapy to shrink a tumor. Touch therapy is a less invasive therapy with virtually no risk. Chemotherapy and radiation therapy can provide both treatment of the cancer and reduction of pain. **Bony metastases** are often very painful because of the bone destruction they cause; radiation is frequently used for this type of pain. Chemotherapy will also hopefully cause the tumor to shrink, which can relieve pressure on surrounding nerves. However, when these treatments fail to control the pain, the patient will need to look for alternative measures.

Various treatments can be considered for cancer pain, and entire medical textbooks have been written about the many options that exist. In this chapter, we will provide a cursory overview of the more common treatments for some of the more common types of cancer pain.

## Oral Medications

The judicious and appropriate use of various oral medications is the cornerstone of cancer pain treatment. The primary treatment is with a combination of opioid or narcotic pain medications and other medications that work hand-in-hand with traditional pain medications. A physician may use **anti-seizure medications (neuroleptics)**, **antidepressants**, anti-inflammatory, and/or other medications to treat cancer pain, especially when there is a neuropathic component (nerve injury or nerve damage). In other words, your doctor may use narcotic pain medication to treat your bone and soft-tissue pain while using other medications to treat associated nerve damage. **Anti-inflammatories** can sometimes help, especially with **metastatic bone cancer**, because they inhibit prostaglandin release, which is associated with bone pain. Unfortunately, many of these medications have side effects, especially at the dosages required to treat cancer pain. When intolerable side effects such as excessive sedation, confusion, constipation, and nausea occur or inadequate pain treatment is noted, referral to an interventional pain specialist may provide other more effective solutions.

## Destructive Block Therapy

One of the most common forms of cancer pain treatment done by interventional pain physicians is for pancreatic cancer. Unfortunately, pancreatic cancer usually presents late and generally has a fairly poor prognosis. Patients can suffer from severe abdominal pain that is often not adequately managed with pain medications. A specific group of nerves, the **celiac plexus**, sits behind the **pancreas**; these **innervate** the pancreas and much of the other surrounding viscera (abdominal organs). Blockade of this group of nerves can provide profound pain relief when the pain is coming from the pancreas or other adjacent abdominal (visceral) structures. Physicians may choose to first perform a diagnostic local anesthetic injection to prove that it results in symptomatic relief and later perform a **neurolytic** (nerve-killing) injection to destroy the celiac nerves to decrease the patient's ability to feel that particular organ. Some physicians will choose to proceed directly to the neurolytic injection (after appropriate discussion with the patient) to avoid the need for multiple treatments, especially when ongoing chemotherapy and other treatments are required.

This treatment is highly effective for abdominal pain associated with pancreatic cancer and other upper abdominal tumors. However, when pancreatic cancer causes back pain, this treatment may not be as effective. Back pain from this type of cancer is often caused by erosion of the pancreatic tumor into the back muscles, and that requires an alternative type of treatment, typically with **neuraxial (spinal) narcotic medications** (please see chapter 20).

There are many other nerves in the body that can be blocked for prolonged periods of time to treat cancer pain. These therapies usually require a **diagnostic injection** of the target nerve with local anesthetic to determine whether this is a viable option for treatment of the cancer-related pain. (Celiac plexus blocks are so predictable that some physicians will bypass this step with that type of block.) Peripheral nerve blocks can treat many different cancer-related pain syndromes, especially those involving the abdominal wall or extremity. Rectal pain may respond to blockade of the **ganglion impar.** The number of different nerves that can be blocked to assist with cancer pain management is beyond the scope of this book.

## Spinal Narcotics

Metastases to bone and primary bone tumors often can cause severe pain that may or may not respond to maximal doses of radiation. When pain persists in these regions and isn't adequately controlled by oral or transdermal (through the skin) pain medications, some consideration should be given to spinal narcotics. Several techniques are available, and the patient's life expectancy will often guide the clinician's choice of which technique to utilize. This may sound rather cold and clinical, but it is really a consideration guided by the recovery time related to these procedures, the associated costs, and providing the best quality of life for the patient.

Two basic techniques are used to provide spinal narcotics: a **catheter** placed into the **epidural space** or the **subarachnoid space** (called an **intrathecal drug delivery system**). The first modality is most appropriate for someone with a shorter life expectancy because the catheters tend to dislodge, clog, and/or break over longer periods of time and there is a progressively elevated risk of infection the longer they are left in place because these catheters typically exit through the skin to an external pump. However they require a much less invasive surgery and recovery is almost immediate. Their initial cost is less but with time, (by three to four months) they can become less cost effective due to the higher ongoing maintenance costs.

The second modality is a more permanent version and is used in patients with a life expectancy of four to six months or greater. It is a more invasive procedure that requires more involved surgery and an overnight hospital admission. The pump itself is very expensive (about $20,000), and some insurance companies will not cover the pump for patients who have a life expectancy of less than six months. If your oncologist has given you a six-month life expectancy, you need to decide how you want to live those last six months. Be honest with your physicians. If you want to travel for as long as possible, then an external pump will likely not be an option due to the need for frequent nursing care, and even an implantable pump could be difficult unless you plan to be around for refills (usually once every month or two). You may prefer the freedom of oral medications. For more detailed information on spinal narcotic treatment, see chapter 20.

Cancer pain management is something that no one wants to talk about because it isn't a cure for the disease. The driving focus of cancer treatment is destroying the cancer so the individual can lead a long and healthy life. Sometimes the treatment for this disease causes **chronic pain**, which in turn needs to be treated. In the most severe cases, pain management physicians are brought in to give the terminal patient the best possible quality of life for their remaining days. Whatever the situation, it is important to have a realistic goal for treatment. Pain control is about maximizing your quality of life while avoiding unwanted side effects and the need for more frequent physician visits. Improved pain control has been associated with improved length of survival. Successful treatment of cancer pain is about communication between you, your family, your oncologist, and your pain management physician.

## Questions to Ask Your Physician:

1. What is my long-term prognosis?

2. What are my treatment goals? For example, if you have been given a six-month life expectancy, how do you want to spend those six months? Is it important to travel? Be cognitively intact? Be at home with family and friends?

3. What kind of treatment am I pursuing with my oncologist— curative or **palliative** (treating symptoms but not changing the end result)? Your pain management treatment and oncology treatments must be coordinated, as some treatments can't be given at the same time.

# CHAPTER 22

## INSURANCE: COPAYS, COINSURANCE, DEDUCTIBLES, OH MY!

Health insurance is a particularly tricky system to navigate. Policies change rapidly, leaving patients in shock when procedures or tests they believed would be covered are not. There was a time when you would go to your doctor's office, pay your **copay**, and everything would be fine. Today we live in a world of insurance policies that require varying amounts of patient responsibility. This responsibility is not just financial. It isn't enough to know how much your copay is; you must know who participates with your plan before you make an appointment or if you need a primary care physician referral. The purpose of this chapter is to demystify some of the insurance language that is casually spoken at your doctor's office and to help you better understand your benefits.

The first point that must be made is your health insurance is your responsibility. When you signed up for your health insurance plan, you were probably given a booklet explaining your plan and your benefits. It's a lot of information thrown at you very quickly. If you have any questions about what is covered, which doctors participate in your plan, or what your financial responsibility is, call your insurer at the phone number on the back of your insurance card. This line is staffed with professionals who are trained to help you understand your coverage. Remember to write down the name of the person you spoke to, as well as the date and time you spoke to them. If there is ever any question about the information you received, you must be able to prove you made this phone call. Patients often believe that calling their insurance company is a job best left to the professionals in their doctor's office. This is a good place to start, but because you are ultimately responsible for any bills generated from the care you receive, firsthand knowledge from your own conversation with the carrier can be helpful. The people in your doctor's office are very knowledgeable about insurance in general, but they may not know everything about your specific policy. Employers sometimes negotiate specific exclusions to policies to decrease their costs, and only the beneficiary (patient) and the employer are allowed to see these specific details of your policy.

For the rest of this chapter we are going to discuss the various terms that are used to describe insurance. Understanding these terms is a good start to understanding your insurance plan.

## Primary Care Physician Referral

This is a recommendation made by your primary care physician (otherwise known as a general practitioner, family doctor, internist, or PCP) to see a specialist. Many insurance companies require that you obtain a referral before seeing a specialist. This referral can be as simple as a piece of paper with the recommendation on it or as complex as a formal recommendation to your insurance company. The more formal recommendation will specify a number of times you can be seen as well as a date range for care. The formal referral will also have a reference number. If your plan requires the more formal referral, you should be aware of the referral number, the number of visits specified, and the date range for care. If the number of times you are seen exceeds the amount specified by the referral or occurs outside of the date range, you will need to extend or increase the number of visits in the referral, or you may be responsible for the doctor's charge. If you show up at the specialist's office without a referral from your primary care physician, the office may turn you away without being seen. Save yourself time, aggravation, and money by making sure you have a referral in place before your appointment.

## Copays

Many people assume that because the doctor is being paid by the insurance company, he or she can afford to write off your copay, the amount of the doctor's bill for which you are directly responsible. As a point of background, it is likely that your doctor negotiated a contract with your insurance plan so that he or she could be considered a participating provider. The insurance company may have looked at the rate your doctor charges for various procedures and negotiated to pay a percentage of that charge, or alternatively they may have agreed upon an independent fee schedule that was mutually acceptable to both sides, which is called the contracted rate. Your insurance company then decided on a set charge that you are responsible for if you see a specialist, and that's your copay. Your copay is deducted from the amount the insurance carrier agreed to pay your doctor (the contracted rate). If your doctor doesn't collect the copay, he isn't getting paid the full amount of his contracted rate. In addition, most contracts require that the doctor collect this copay or face significant penalties. Yes, your doctor can actually get in trouble for not taking your copay. Remember, he or she signed a contract with your insurance company guaranteeing that he would collect this fee, and violating the contract can have severe repercussions for the doctor.

Not all copays are the same. The front of your card may list the amount of your copay for seeing a primary care physician or a specialist. There may also be other copays that you don't see on the front of the card. For example, you may have a $500 copay for outpatient surgery. You have to pay this copay every time you have an outpatient procedure done. You may also have a higher copay for procedures that require an overnight stay at the hospital. Knowing your copays ahead of time can save you a lot of time and aggravation. If you know your copay, you will know if you are in a financial position to afford a procedure. Some procedures can be performed at the doctor's office for a much lower copay (office copay instead of an outpatient surgery copay). This means (in most cases) that you won't be able to get intravenous sedation, but many people would rather be uncomfortable for a few minutes than pay the larger copay; your doctor can help guide you as to what procedures might require some sedation.

## Deductibles and Coinsurance

Some insurance plans don't have copays. Instead, they use **deductibles** and coinsurance as a means of passing back to you the amount of money you're responsible to pay. Your deductible is a set amount of money that you have to pay out before your insurance company pays any of the bill. For example, if you have a $1,000 deductible, your doctor will submit his or her charges and the insurance company will send you an Explanation of Benefits (EOB) telling you what portion of the bill you are responsible to pay.

Your doctor's office will get a copy of the same EOB and mail you a bill reflecting the money owed. This balance is not the doctor's full charge; it is the contracted rate your doctor has with your insurance company. If you have not met your deductible then you are responsible for these bills. The benefit to this type of plan (over trying to negotiate a rate with your doctor on your own) is that your insurance company has already gotten you a significantly reduced rate as they have negotiated on behalf of all the members of your plan. You doctor was willing to take less money from the company in exchange for the increase in volume of patients he can see as a participating provider. Today High-Deductible Plans are becoming ever more popular; in this situation, the patient is responsible often for at least the first $2,000 and sometimes up to $10,000 depending on the plan. Patients can often manage these expenses in a tax-efficient fashion using a health savings account or flexible health spending account.

Once you have reached your deductible, your insurance company may pick up 100 % or you may be responsible for coinsurance. This is the percentage of money you are responsible for paying until you reach your **out-of-pocket maximum** for the year. For example, let's imagine that you go to see your doctor after your deductible has been met. At this point, you are responsible for 20 % coinsurance: on a $100 charge, they will pay $80 and you will pay $20. They will send you an EOB in the mail telling you they paid the $80 they're responsible for and you must now pay the $20. Most plans have a cap on how much they expect you to pay every year. This cap is called your out-of-pocket maximum. Some plans include your deductible in the out-of-pocket maximum and others do not. This is a good question to ask your insurance company so you have a realistic idea of how much money you will have to pay. High-deductible plans have become very popular over the last several years, especially in the form of health savings accounts (HSAs) or flexible health spending accounts. All of these have the goal of controlling the employer's health care costs, unfortunately, usually at the expense of shifting these costs to you, the patient. If you think this is all about shifting more and more expenses to you the patient, then you have figured out the game; congratulations.

## Questions to Ask Before Your First Appointment:

1. Does the doctor participate with my insurance plan?
2. Do I need a primary care physician referral?
3. Do I have a copay when I see a specialist? If so, what is the copay?
4. What is my copay for outpatient surgery?
5. Do I have a deductible or coinsurance?

# CHAPTER 23

---

## WORKERS'COMPENSATION: HOW IT WORKS AND WHAT TO DO IF IT DOESN'T

$I$f you were injured on the job or your pain is related to repetitive-motion activity at work, then you may find yourself dealing with your state's workers' compensation system. If you are not frustrated yet, you likely will be soon.

The workers' compensation system can be difficult and aggravating for both you and your physician, to say the least. There are multiple obstacles that can derail or limit your care. You and your physician will need to deal with the insurance company, attorneys, state rules, **adjusters, case managers,** and many other layers between you and your health care. Unfortunately, this only adds another level of complexity to the care of patients with **chronic pain.** Some physicians have far more experience with workers' compensation care and understand the system, which can help the patient navigate through the quicksand. Workers' compensation has historically resisted and limited pain management to **claimants** (injured workers). Your initial treatment, and even surgeries, may have been approved with little delay (although possibly not), but don't be surprised if your care comes to a grinding halt when chronic pain treatments become necessary.

The workers' compensation system was federally legislated in 1906 and was an insurance instituted to protect employers from lawsuits arising from injuries that occurred on the job. It was designed to provide a system for injured workers to receive health care while limiting the employer's exposure. Workers' compensation was intended to provide care to workers and hold the employer responsible for the injury, both for health care as well as any settlement for long-term damage. However, as you know, whenever money is involved, there are bound to be conflicts at multiple levels.

To be fair, the problem is not workers' compensation alone. Unfortunately, some claimants (injured workers and/or their physicians) have previously "gamed the system" to take advantage of insurance carriers and their employers. As the saying goes, a few can ruin it for the many. Because of this, the rules and regulations surrounding workers' compensation have grown increasingly complex and more difficult. Despite this cynical outlook, many carriers, case managers, adjusters, and workers' compensation programs truly care about their patients and will help them to get better and return to work. However, if yours is not one of them, you might be in for a long ride.

Workers' compensation has multiple levels of complexity. We will provide a general description of workers' compensation systems, but each state sets up its own rules and regulations to govern their individual systems and your doctor and/or attorney should be able to provide you with additional guidance. Below are common terms that you should be familiar with.

*Claimant:* You, the patient.

*Respondent:* The legal term for your workers' compensation carrier.

*Case manager:* A nurse or other trained health care professional assigned to your case to hopefully help expedite and coordinate your care. He or she should be able to explain to the adjuster what type of treatment your doctor is recommending and why it's a good idea.

*Adjuster:* Often someone with little to no medical knowledge who works for the insurance carrier and is responsible for making your health care coverage decisions. Adjusters also pay your doctor's and pharmacy bills and manage other weekly compensation you may receive while you are out of work.

*Medical director:* A physician who works for the insurance company and helps to oversee their medical policies. He or she will often make medical decisions about more complicated or expensive therapies.

*Peer-to-peer review:* This is supposed to be an "independent" physician's review of the requested treatment and is based on information sent by the carrier to the reviewing physician. This is frequently arranged through a third party company that provides this type of review service and which contracts with doctors to provide this review service. In most peer-to-peer reviews, they are supposed to talk with your doctor over the phone before making a coverage decision. Unfortunately, this process is fraught with problems. Often the reviewer is not given the full extent of information from the carrier in order to make a proper decision. It is sometimes impossible to connect with the other doctor due to conflicting schedules between your doctor and the reviewer, who may be anywhere in the country. Another major problem is that doctors are told they must use specific guidelines, even if not recognized by your particular state, and these guidelines and reviews are therefore often biased toward denial. The company that is hired tracks their denial rate and uses that information to sell their services to the various insurance carriers. These reviews present an inherent conflict of interest: a doctor that approves too much may not be asked to continue doing reviews.

*IME (independent medical examiner):* A physician selected by your insurance company to evaluate your condition. This is usually a face-to-face meeting with a doctor that has been hired by your insurance company as a second opinion. Unfortunately, many insurance carriers have a pool of physicians whom they hire as "independent" medical examiners because of their known biased opinions against certain pain management treatments. Because the IME is selected and paid for by the workers' compensation carrier, he or she is almost never unbiased. Again, if they approve too much, they are often not asked to do more evaluations.

*Commissioner examiner:* A physician assigned by the workers' compensation commissioner to evaluate your case, theoretically a completely neutral physician. While this is not always the case, it is about as fair as that process will ever get.

(Note: Theoretically, neither a commissioner examiner nor an independent medical examiner should subsequently become your treating physician because of the potential for conflict of interest.)

*Workers' compensation hearing:* Each state has its own hearing structure and format. Hearings can be of many types. Informal hearings are those in which the parties gather to discuss obstacles to care and/or payment to the claimant in a nonbinding format. Formal hearings in most states are court-like procedures and have binding decisions associated with them. Unfortunately, it can often take months to schedule these hearings and have a final decision rendered.

When requesting treatment, your physician must provide appropriate letters of medical necessity to workers' compensation that describe your condition and the reasons for the treatment they're recommending. These reports should be typed and sent to your carrier to obtain the necessary approval. Your physician may be required to speak to another physician on the phone to gain approval or authorization (a **peer-to-peer review**). Your physician's staff will likely have to call the carrier, at least once and perhaps 20 times, to get approval or authorization for your treatment. You and your attorney may also need to get involved.

Your attorney should be responsible for helping guide you through the legal aspects of the process. If your carrier cooperates with your care, you may not need an attorney to complete your treatment under workers' compensation. If, however, you experience repetitive delays or just frank denial of treatment, then consider hiring an attorney to assist you through the workers' compensation process. Your attorney will typically be paid from a percentage of your settlement and/or other decisions. Unfortunately, once you hire an attorney in the workers' compensation system it is usually extremely difficult to switch to a new attorney if the first one is not working out. Be careful to hire an attorney who cares about your medical treatment and understands the system. He or she needs to protect your rights to receive medical treatment, not just his or her right to receive a portion of your payment/settlement.

**NOTE:** Some of the above terms, as well as the exact laws, will vary from state to state but the general principles are similar.

# CONCLUSION

In this book we have tried to explain the basics regarding chronic pain, including its causes and treatments. Understanding many of the treatments that are available requires some basic understanding of anatomy; if you have had trouble following some of the treatments, we urge you to go back and at least look through some of the pertinent sections within the anatomy chapter (chapter 4).

Perhaps most importantly, we have tried to educate you in how to identify a physician who has the training and expertise to get to the root of your problem. Today, highly specialized pain medicine physicians exist to expertly and carefully identify the cause of your symptoms. Interventional pain management is a subspecialty of pain medicine that uses precision-guided fluoroscopic injections to both help determine (diagnose) the precise cause of pain and to assist in its treatment.

Most pain conditions can be treated and the symptoms eased. Pain management rarely means pain cure, but rather refers to the long-term management of the condition to minimize the effects on normal activities of daily living. Realistic expectations are essential to an outcome that satisfies both the patient and the doctor.

Future editions of this book will update advances that have occurred in treatment and the understanding of these various diseases. Please feel free to provide us with comments about how we can improve this book in subsequent editions.

# GLOSSARY

**Note:** All Glossary terms are marked in **bold** throughout the text for easy reference.

**Acupuncture:** This is a traditional form of Chinese medicine that involves placing very small needles into the body along certain lines of energy (meridians) to treat a multitude of health conditions, including pain.

**Acupuncturist:** A physician specializing in the use of acupuncture for treatment.

**Adhesiolysis:** A procedure to break up scar tissue that has formed around nerves in the spinal canal.

**Adipose tissue:** The fatty tissue of the body.

**Adjuster:** An employee of a workers' compensation insurance carrier who helps to process and administer the claim and is usually responsible for deciding whether a treatment is approved. Adjusters are typically not nurses or health care professionals and have limited clinical knowledge.

**Adrenaline:** A natural stimulant released by the adrenal gland and other nerve endings in the body to stimulate certain body functions. Release is typically increased in response to stress.

**Agonist:** A drug or chemical that stimulates a specific receptor to cause a desired effect. An agonist will cause the cell to perform the same function that the stimulated nerve receptor would normally initiate.

**Ankylosing spondylitis:** A type of arthritis or connective tissue disorder that affects specific joints of the body and, more specifically, the sacroiliac joints and other parts of the spine.

**Androgenic steroids:** Male hormones such as testosterone.

**Anesthesiologist:** A doctor who has been trained in the field of anesthesia.

**Annulus:** The outer wall of a spinal disc, made up of fibers that circle and strengthen the disc. An intact annulus helps to constrain the nucleus (or center of the disc) from leaking or herniating (pushing out).

**Antagonist:** A drug or chemical that counteracts or inhibits the action at a receptor. This would prevent or decrease the cell's ability to perform the function that this receptor normally causes.

**Anterior:** Towards the front side of the body.

**Anti-anxiety medications (anxiolytics):** Medications that reduce or control anxiety.

**Anticonvulsants:** Medications that stabilize nerve membranes and treat nerve pain, also used for the treatment of seizures.

**Antidepressants:** Medications used in the treatment of depression.

**Anti-inflammatories:** Medications used to treat inflammation, such as is seen with arthritis.

**Anti-seizure medicines:** Medications that work in the same way as anticonvulsants to stabilize nerve membranes and treat nerve pain, particularly used for the treatment of seizures.

**Aorta:** The largest artery of the body. This vessel comes off of the heart and all the remaining arteries are fed from this large vessel as it travels through the chest and abdomen.

**Arrhythmias:** Abnormal heart rhythm (heart beat).

**Arthralgia:** Joint pain and usually implying involvement of more than one joint. Does not indicate the cause of pain but rather it is a term that is descriptive as to the quality of pain.

**Arthroscopy:** Direct visualization with a device that allows the physician to look inside a joint.

**Atlanto-axial (AA) joints:** Paired joints (one on each side) between the top two vertebrae of the spine.

**Atlanto-occipital (AO) joints:** Paired joints (one on each side) between the base of the skull and the first vertebra of the spine.

**Atlas:** The first vertebra of the spine.

**Auriculotemporal nerve:** A nerve that supplies sensation to the area around the ear and temple.

**Axis:** The second vertebra of the spine.

**Baclofen:** An antispasmodic medication commonly used in the treatment of multiple sclerosis and injuries associated with muscle spasm.

**Behavioral counseling:** Psychological counseling that is used to modify behaviors that are abnormal and are contributing to the perpetuation of pain.

**Biacuplasty®:** A heated-needle treatment used for pain that is caused by an abnormal and painful disc.

**"Blind" injections:** An injection done without radiologic guidance.

**Blood thinners:** Medications that are used to keep the blood from clotting in a patient with a history of excessive clotting.

**Bone scan:** A nuclear medicine test that involves the injection of radioactive-labeled material to detect active areas of bone remodeling in the presence of an acute fracture, infection, or arthritis.

**Bony metastasis:** Cancer that has spread from its primary location to the bone.

**Botulinum toxin:** More widely recognized as Botox®. This is a synthetic drug that is injected into muscles to provide prolonged muscle relaxation.

**Brachial plexus:** The collection of nerves that supply the arm with motor function and sensation.

**Bupivacaine:** A long-acting local anesthetic.

**Cardiologist:** A doctor who specializes in treating heart conditions.

**Cannula:** A hollow tube used by doctors for medical treatments. These tubes come in many different sizes ranging from tiny to large.

**C-arm:** An x-ray machine that allows the doctor to take live pictures while they work. The "C-arm" allows the doctor to rotate the direction that an image is taken to provide multiple views and angles of the area under study. In continuous mode, it can allow the doctor to see the movement of needles or dye within the body. This is used to perform most spinal injections.

**Carpal bones:** Bones of the wrist and base of hand.

**Case manager:** Usually a nurse or other health care professional that works for an insurance company to help coordinate care and improve communication and efficiency of treatment.

**CAT scan (CT scan):** A type of x-ray machine that takes multiple images and then, via computer programming, summates the images to provide specific and special views of the body. Standard CT provides two-dimensional information regarding the anatomy of structures. Recent advances now allow for 3D reconstruction using CT imaging.

**Catheter:** A hollow tube that doctors use to deliver fluid/medication or, in some circumstances, drain fluid from an area of the body.

**Catheter tip granuloma:** A fibrous nodule or scar tissue that forms around the tip of a spinal catheter.

**Caudal epidural injections:** An injection into the epidural space inside the tailbone (sacrum).

**Causalgia:** Nerve pain that arises specifically from damaged peripheral nerves.

**Celiac plexus:** A group of nerves within the abdomen that provides nerve supply and feeling for the liver, pancreas, and much of the intestines. This nerve is frequently destroyed by injecting chemicals in the treatment of cancer pain from abdominal organs to decrease the sensation (feeling) coming from that area of the body.

**Central nervous system:** The brain and spinal cord (as opposed to the peripheral nervous system, which is outside the brain and spine).

**Cervical vertebrae:** Spinal bones of the neck.

**Chemotherapy:** Medications used to treat cancer and certain rheumatologic conditions.

**Chiropractor:** A doctor who specializes in manipulation of joints and the spine to bring structures back into normal alignment, thereby treating pain.

**Chronic pain:** Pain that has been present for more than two or three months, or beyond the expected length of healing.

**Claimant:** An injured worker who has made a claim for disability compensation or health care benefits from a workers compensation insurance company.

**Cluneal nerve:** A nerve that supplies sensation in the buttock region.

**Coccyx:** The tailbone.

**Commissioners' exam:** An exam ordered by the judge or commissioner in a workers' compensation case. Typically performed by an independent physician.

**Complex regional pain syndrome (CRPS):** A disorder characterized by hyperactivity of the nervous system that usually arises from a nerve injury. It is often a particularly painful condition that can severely interrupt normal lifestyle.

**"Contained" herniation:** A disc herniation that has not broken through the outer wall (annulus) of the disc.

**Copayment (copay):** The patient's portion of payment, usually a specific dollar amount, which will be billed repeatedly until the patient reaches their out-of-pocket maximum for the year.

**Cryoneuroablation:** A procedure that freezes peripheral nerves to treat pain.

**Deductible:** The patient's payment responsibility, which must be met before the insurance carrier will begin to make any payments.

**Deep peroneal nerve:** A nerve that supplies sensation and motor function to the calf and foot.

**Degeneration:** Natural aging process.

**Diagnostic injection:** An injection of local anesthetic (numbing medication) that helps to document the cause of pain. A positive response suggests that the structure is causing pain, whereas a negative response suggests it is not.

**Diaphragm:** The main breathing muscle of the body. This also separates the abdomen from the chest internally.

**Digital nerves:** Nerves that supply sensation to the fingers and toes.

**Discs:** The shock absorbers between the bones of the spine.

**Disc decompression:** A procedure that decreases the pressure inside of the disc and is used to remove a disc herniation or protrusion.

**Disc herniation (disc bulge):** A disc that protrudes or sticks out abnormally and which usually causes pain by pushing on, or touching, a nerve; looks like a bubble on the side wall of a tire.

**Discitis:** An infection of the disc, a very serious condition that requires immediate attention.

**Discogenic pain:** Pain that arises from the intervertebral disc usually associated with a torn, protruding, and/or degenerated disc.

**Discogram:** A diagnostic test that allows the physician to determine if a particular disc is painful by applying progressively increasing pressure through a needle to the center of the disc (see chapter 16 for a full description of this diagnostic test).

**Disc tear:** A crack or tear of the outer wall (annulus) of the disc, which can allow material to escape from the center of the disc.

**Dry needling:** A procedure in which a needle is placed in the body without the injection of medication. A technique for trigger point injections– typically used for the treatment of painful muscle spots.

**Edema:** Swelling from accumulation of fluid in body tissues.

**Electrocardiogram (ECG):** A basic test that looks at the electrical function of the heart.

**Electrodiagnostic testing:** A general term that describes a variety of tests that look at the function of nerves.

**Electromyography (EMG):** An electrical test that looks at whether muscles are receiving normal nerve supply.

**Electrostimulation:** The stimulation of nerves and muscles.

**Epidural blood patch:** The injection of blood into the epidural space for the treatment of a spinal fluid leak (usually created by a needle hole).

**Epidural space:** A potential space in the spine which physicians use to deliver medications to various structures (usually nerves) within the spine.

**Extruded herniation:** A disc herniation that is larger than its base, i.e. mushroom-like in appearance.

**Facet joints:** Paired (one on each side of the body) joints of the spine that exist at each and every spinal level. These joints participate in the motion of the spine.

**Femoral nerve:** One of the two main nerves of the lower extremity (sciatic is the other).

**Fibroblasts:** Cells within the body that make up the basic structure of tissue and which are frequently involved in remodeling of injuries.

**Fluoroscopic guidance:** The physician uses live x-ray pictures to guide his treatment.

**Foot drop:** A condition caused by nerve injury in the leg or back, resulting in the foot flopping down when walking. Patients commonly need a brace to prevent tripping and falling.

**Ganglia:** A collection of nerve cells.

**Ganglion impar:** A collection of nerve cells that lie in front of the tailbone and sacrum.

**Genitofemoral nerve:** A nerve that supplies the groin and scrotal or labial region with sensation.

**Glucocorticosteroids:** A type of steroid that physicians inject to reduce inflammation.

**Histamine:** A chemical that the body releases, usually related to allergic reactions.

**Humerus:** The bone in the upper arm.

**Hypertrophy:** Enlarged or overgrown. As in a joint which is distorted by arthritis.

**Hypogastric plexus:** A group of nerves that lie in front of the spine where it joins the sacrum.

**Independent medical examiner (IME):** An examiner who is expected to objectively evaluate the patient, usually to determine if the treatment the physician prescribes is appropriate and should be covered by the insurance company.

**Intradiscal electrothermal annuloplasty (IDET®):** A procedure that treats pain coming from the disc, related to tears or fissures in the outer wall (annulus).

**Infraorbital nerve:** A nerve that supplies sensation to facial structures below the eye and above the jaw.

**Infrapatellar saphenous nerve:** A nerve that runs along the inside of the knee and that is most frequently damaged during knee surgery. This nerve supplies sensory function to the front of the knee.

**Injectate:** A substance to be injected into the body.

**Innervate:** To supply nerve feeling to an area.

**Insulin:** A natural or synthetic compound that helps the body control metabolism of sugars.

**Intercostal nerve:** A nerve that runs under the rib and that supplies sensation to the chest wall.

**Interstitial cystitis:** A condition affecting the bladder that can cause severe pain. Some experts think this is analogous to complex regional pain syndrome (CRPS) of the bladder.

**Interventional pain management (IPM):** The treatment of pain using injection and surgical techniques.

**Intra-articular injection:** An injection made inside the joint.

**Intradiscal techniques:** Procedures that treat the disc by operating inside the disc.

**Intrathecal drug delivery system:** A device that delivers medication into the spinal fluid, usually on a continuous basis.

**Ischemic compression (acupressure):** A treatment that is similar to acupuncture, but uses pressure on acupuncture points and trigger points.

**Laser assisted spinal endoscopy (LASE):** A device that removes disc material through a cannula, under direct visualization and with the assistance of a laser.

**Lateral:** Toward the left or right side of the body.

**Lateral calcaneal nerve:** A sensory nerve around the outside of the heel.

**Lateral epicondylitis:** Also known as 'tennis elbow,' this is a condition characterized by pain and tenderness along the outside of the elbow.

**Lateral recess:** An area inside the spinal canal that is off to the side. The disc lies anterior and the facet joint lies posterior to this region.

**Leaking disc:** A disc with a tear that goes through the entire outer wall (annulus) and allows chemicals within the disc to leak out. These chemicals usually cause irritation or inflammation of the surrounding structures.

**Ligament:** Tissue that connects one bone to another bone, providing stability of joints.

**Ligament flavum:** A ligament that runs along the back of the spinal canal and which physicians use to help them identify the epidural space. Overgrowth of this ligament can cause spinal stenosis.

**Local anesthetic phase:** A medication that is injected to numb the area or nerve.

**Long-acting opioid:** Pain medications with a sustained-release formula to reduce the frequency with which pills must be taken.

**Lumbar vertebral bones:** Bones of the spine in the lower back.

**Medial branch block (MBB):** Injection of local anesthetic and steroids onto the nerves of the facets.

**Medial calcaneal nerve:** A sensory nerve that lies along the inside of the heel.

**Medical marijuana:** The use of marijuana for medicinal purposes.

**Mental nerve:** A nerve that exits through the lower jaw (the mandible) and which supplies sensation to the skin and soft tissues over the jaw.

**Metastases:** Cancer that has spread to areas of the body beyond where the cancer started.

**Metastatic bone cancer:** Cancer that has spread to bone.

**Mineralocorticoid steroids:** A steroid that influences salt and water balance in the body.

**Morton's neuroma:** an overgrown bundle of nerves in the foot, usually between the third and fourth toes.

**Myelogram:** A diagnostic test that involves the injection of dye into the spinal canal to identify areas of nerve compression.

**Myofascial pain syndrome:** Pain that involves the muscles and causes trigger points.

**Neural foramen:** A hole or space in the spine between spinal levels (bones) where nerves exit.

**Neuraxial medications:** Medications that are delivered directly into the spinal fluid.

**Neurologist:** A doctor who specializes in conditions affecting nerves.

**Neurolytic:** A medication or chemical that destroys nerves.

**Neurosurgeon:** A physician who specializes in operating on the brain and spine.

**Nerve conduction study (NCS):** A test that measures how well nerves conduct impulses in the body (see chapter 5)

**Nucleoplasty®:** A treatment that is performed through a needle to decompress a disc herniation.

**Nucleotome®:** A treatment that decompresses a disc herniation via a small hollow tube.

**Nucleus:** The center of a structure.

**Nucleus pulposus:** The center of the vertebral disc.

**Occipital nerve:** A nerve that supplies sensation to the back and top of the skull.

**Occiput:** The back and base of the skull.

**Oncology:** The treatment and study of cancer.

**Orthopedist:** A physician who specializes in the surgical and non-surgical treatment of bone and joint injuries.

**Orthotics:** A device that is placed in the shoe to restore normal alignment.

**Out-of-pocket maximum:** The maximum amount of money that a patient (or family) must pay for health care in one year.

**Palliative treatment:** Treatments that help relieve symptoms but do not cure the problem.

**Palpation:** To feel with the fingers to identify a problem.

**Pancreas:** An organ in the abdomen that secretes chemicals and hormones to assist with digestion and blood sugar control.

**Pancreatitis:** Inflammation or irritation of the pancreas, usually caused by alcohol, drugs, or a blockage of the outflow of digestive enzymes.

**Patella:** Knee cap. This bone slides over the knee as the joint moves.

**Peer-to-peer review:** When one doctor with a similar expertise reviews the work of another doctor to determine the appropriateness of treatment. This often involves a conversation between the treating and reviewing physician.

**Percutaneous:** A procedure performed through the skin, without cutting open the body.

**Percutaneous endoscopic discectomies:** A procedure in which a disc is removed without a surgical incision.

**Peripheral nerves:** Nerves outside the spinal canal.

**Periscapular:** Between the shoulder blades

**Peritonitis:** An infection of the abdominal cavity.

**Peroneal nerve:** A nerve that starts behind the knee and runs down the outside of the leg to the foot and which provides both motor function and sensation to the leg.

**Phantom-limb pain:** Pain that is sensed by the patient in a structure (usually an arm or leg) that has been lost or amputated.

**Phenol:** A chemical that is injected to destroy nerves and treat pain; usually reserved for the treatment of cancer pain. It is also used to treat chronic muscular spasm by injecting at motor endpoints.

**Physiatrist:** A physician who specializes in the treatment and rehabilitation of the body.

**Piriformis muscle:** The muscle in the buttock which lies on top of the sciatic nerve and helps move the leg outwards.

**Plantar fasciitis:** Inflammation or irritation of the bottom of the foot which can cause severe pain with walking.

**Pneumothorax:** Collapse of the lung, usually caused by trauma to the lung surface as when struck by a needle (like a balloon with a hole, the air will leak out and the balloon collapses).

**Posterior:** Towards the back side of the body.

**Postdural puncture headaches:** Headaches that are caused by the leak of spinal fluid, usually following insertion of a needle into the spinal fluid.

**Posterior joint syndrome:** Pain coming from both the lumbar facet and sacroiliac joints.

**Prophylactic antibiotics:** Antibiotics that are given to help prevent infection.

**Pseudoradicular symptoms:** Symptoms that radiate into the extremity, but are not caused by nerve compression in the spinal canal.

**Pseudosciatica:** Similar to pseudoradicular symptoms, although Pseudosciatica specifically refers to such pain in the leg.

**Psoriatic arthritis:** An arthritic condition that is associated with psoriasis and can affect multiple joints of the body, but commonly involves the sacroiliac joint.

**Radial nerve:** A nerve that supplies sensation and motor function to parts of the arm and hand.

**Radiation neuritis:** Irritation or damage of nerves from radiation, commonly seen following cancer treatments.

**Radiculopathy:** Pain from a nerve that is irritated or compressed inside the spinal canal or as it exits the spinal canal.

**Radiofrequency ablation (RFA):** Use of electrical energy to kill nerves.

**Rectus abdominus:** Vertical abdominal muscles that run from the breastbone to the pelvis. Also known as the "six-pack".

**Referred pain:** Pain that is sensed by the patient in an area that is removed (away) from the area of injury.

**Reiter's syndrome:** Also known as reactive arthritis, this condition is a form of inflammatory arthritis.

**Retro-orbital:** Behind the eyes.

**Respiratory depression:** Decreased breathing drive or decreased rate of breathing; as can occur with drug overdose.

**Sacroiliac joint:** A joint of the pelvis between the iliac bone and sacrum.

**Sacroiliitis:** Inflammation of the sacroiliac joint.

**Saphenous nerve:** A nerve that runs along the inside of the thigh and calf, ending in the foot, and which supplies sensation to these parts of the leg.

**Sciatica:** A generic term used by many people to mean different things. "True sciatica" involves irritation of the sciatic nerve, but many people incorrectly use this term synonymously with radiculopathy.

**Sciatic nerve:** The largest nerve in the body. This nerve runs from the buttock to behind the knee where it turns into the common peroneal nerve. The sciatic nerve supplies important motor function and sensation to the leg.

**Short-acting opioid:** A narcotic pain medication that typically lasts between three and six hours.

**Spinal canal:** The hole or tube that runs inside the spine from the skull to the sacrum and contains the spinal cord, nerves, and spinal fluid.

**Spinal decompression therapy:** A physical medicine treatment that places traction on the spine to treat disorders of the spine.

**Spinal drug delivery system:** A device that infuses medications into the spinal fluid.

**Spinal stenosis:** Narrowing of the spinal canal; commonly caused by the overgrowth of bone or ligaments around the spine.

**Spondylolisthesis:** A condition where one bone of the spine slips on top of the other so that they are no longer in proper alignment.

**Stellate ganglion:** A group of nerves that supplies specialized nerve function (autonomic sympathetic nerves) to the upper quadrant of the body (arm and face on one side).

**Stem cells:** Cells that can differentiate into multiple different types of tissue in the body.

**Subarachnoid:** The space inside the spinal canal where the spinal fluid, nerves, and spinal cord reside.

**Superior gluteal nerve:** A nerve that supplies sensation to the buttocks.

**Supraorbital nerve:** A nerve that supplies sensation to the area over the eyes (the forehead).

**Suprascapular nerve:** A nerve that supplies some of the shoulder muscles with motor function. This nerve is also felt to have some pain sensation properties.

**Superficial peroneal nerve:** A nerve that supplies sensation to the inside, top of the foot.

**Sympathetic nerves:** A part of the autonomic nervous system that controls functions such as sweating and blood vessel caliber. This system is activated in the fight-or-flight response.

**Synthetic opioid:** An opioid that does not exist in nature, but is created by pharmaceutical manufacturing.

**Tendonitis:** A condition characterized by inflammation of the tendon.

**Transcutaneous electrical nerve stimulation (TENS) units:** A variety of topical electrical stimulating devices.

**Transitional segments:** An abnormal connection of the spine and sacrum where there are too many or too few lumbar spinal bones.

**Ultrasound:** A device that looks into the body using ultrasound waves. Reflection of the waves off of tissue are measured by the device and converted into images, allowing the physician to look at soft tissues and nerves without radiation exposure.

**Ulnar nerve:** One of the nerves that supplies the arm and hand with sensation and motor function, including the ring and pinky fingers.

**Vasoconstriction:** A condition in which a blood vessel narrows, decreasing the amount of blood flow to the area that it supplies.

**Vasomotor changes:** Changes in the appearance of an extremity that are caused by changes in blood flow. Increased flow makes the area red and hot, while decreased flow makes it pale and cold.

**Wet tap (dural puncture):** When an epidural needle accidentally penetrates the dura, this can cause a spinal headache if too much spinal fluid leaks from the hole.

**Zygapophyseal joints:** Paired joints (one on each side) that separate each vertebral bone from the next (except between the first and second vertebral bodies). Movement at the spinal level occurs at these joints.

# ONLINE RESOURCES

**American Chronic Pain Association (ACPA)**
(www.theacpa.org)
This site helps facilitate peer support and education for individuals with chronic pain and their families so that these individuals may live more fully in spite of their pain.

**American Pain Foundation**
(www.painfoundation.org)
Founded in 1997, the American Pain Foundation (APF) is an independent nonprofit organization that serves people affected by pain. APF speaks out for people living with pain, caregivers, health care providers and allied organizations, working together to dismantle the barriers that impede access to quality pain care for all. The American Pain Foundation educates, supports, and advocates for people affected by pain.

**American Society of Interventional Pain Physicians (ASIPP)**
(www.asipp.org)
The American Society of Interventional Pain Physicians (ASIPP) was formed in 1998 with the goal of promoting the development and practice of safe, high-quality yet cost-effective interventional pain management techniques for the diagnosis and treatment of pain and related disorders, and to ensure patient access to these interventions. The ASIPP is a not-for-profit organization representing interventional pain physicians across the country.

**Boston Scientific**
(www.controlyourpain.com)
This site provides patients with information on Boston Scientifics' products such as Precision. It also has information on reimbursement for the patient that might be helpful for them as they go forward with an SCS device.

### Medtronic Pain Therapies

(www.tamethepain.com)

This site provides information on Medtronic pain therapies, including patient testimonials, an overview of how neurostimulation therapy works, and answers to commonly asked questions.

### Race Against Pain

(www.raceagainstpain.com)

This Boston Scientific site allows patients to connect with other patients regarding questions on pain and alternatives that have helped others. It is an active forum that, although sponsored by Boston Scientific, is very open about all modalities and companies. The goal is to allow the patients to tell their own story in their own words.

### St. Jude Medical Neuromodulation

(www.poweroveryourpain.com)

This is a patient education website, sponsored by St. Jude Medical, where you can locate an interventional pain physician, request a spinal cord stimulation (SCS) information kit, and watch videos from patients who live with these systems.

# Northport-East Northport Public Library

To view your patron record from a computer, click on
the Library's homepage: www.nenpl.org

You may:
- request an item be placed on hold
- renew an item that is overdue
- view titles and due dates checked out on your card
- view your own outstanding fines

151 Laurel Avenue
Northport, NY 11768
631-261-6930